Basic Hairdressing

A coursebook for Level 2

4th edition

Stephanie Henderson

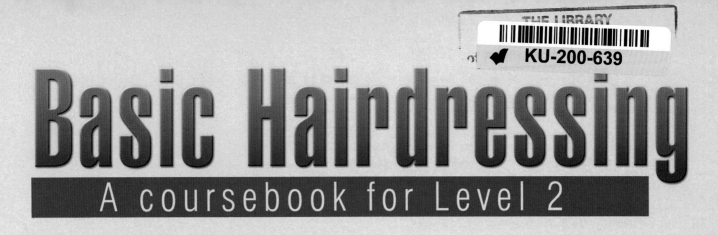

Published in 2003 by:
Nelson Thornes Ltd
Delta Place
27 Bath Road
CHELTENHAM
GL53 7TH
United Kingdom

03 04 05 06 07 / 10 9 8 7 6 5 4 3 2 1

A catalogue record for this book is available from the British Library

ISBN 0 7487 7082 8

Page make-up by IFA Design Ltd, Plymouth, Devon

Printed and bound in Spain by Graficas Estella

Contents

Preface

The Haringtons Salons Group is honoured to have been asked to create the images for the step-by-steps and front cover of the new, updated edition of *Basic Hairdressing* by Stephanie Henderson.

With a dynamic group of seven salons and a staff of 170, Haringtons have a real understanding of every step of the training process. They have their own Internal Education System and NVQ Accredited Training Centre that develops and nurtures young talent, as Haringtons believe that the future of their salons is in the hands of the people they are training today.

As a salon group, they offer full training leading to NVQ Levels 2 and 3 and Key Skills leading to a Modern Apprenticeship. They firmly believe that the people they employ are their greatest asset and that education is where it begins. They are passionate about ongoing staff development and committed to training and ensuring that everyone reaches their full potential.

It is this structure and philosophy, as well having their own International Artistic Team, that made them the ideal choice when looking for a team to organise the photo-shoot and create the inspirational hairstyles and photographic images you can see in the book and on the front cover.

The Artistic Team appears the world over, to inspire, educate and motivate with shows, seminars and workshops that break the boundaries of hairdressing today. Their photographic work pushes the realms of hairdressing creativity while making a statement with images that reflect life on the street and is regularly featured on the front covers and pages of glossy magazines and trade journals internationally. Inspired by everything from music and fashion to art and even architecture, the team is passionate about communicating their interpretations.

It is this passion, together with ground-breaking philosophies and a professional management style, that ensures Haringtons plays a part in driving forward the industry as a whole. They believe that without continued education we cannot develop as an industry and that hairdressers have to feel excited to maintain a progressive environment for their clients.

Haringtons salons @ London, Maidenhead, Marlow, Windsor,
Reading, Beaconsfield and Northwood
www.haringtons.com

Acknowledgments

The author would like to thank a number of people who have helped with the production of this book:

Sharon Williams and Catherine Avadis for their contributions to the text. Francesca Gould for the Indian head massage section.

Haringtons, particularly Lisa Penry, for organising the step-by-step photos used in Chapter 7.
Photographer: Jason Eggby
Make-up: Emily Newsome
Hair: Nick Bland and Darren Bain for Haringtons
Styling: Ziad Ghanem Ltd.

Uxbridge College, for the photographic examples accompanying the text.
Photographer: Martin Sookias
Coordinator: Jo Kearvell
Students: Jenny Adnett, Vanessa Badall, Zeenat Brigden, Chloe Drew, Carrie-Ann Feeney, Claire Fountain, Chris Greaves, Dionne Hallam, Anne Kemp, Alice Liu, Bose Oyebamiji Natasha Pavlovskaia, Rebecca Russell, Lynn Swift, Vicky Waters and M-Ul-Haq.

Photo credits:

- American Dream (p. 153 top)
- Babyliss (p. 125)
- Chubb Fire (p. 60)
- Clynol (p. 130; p. 134; p. 140; p. 149 top; p. 183; p. 193 right)
- Corel 669 (NT) (p. 132)
- Corel 698 (NT) (p. 192; p. 193 left and middle)
- Denman (p. 120; p. 121; p. 165 bottom)
- EWI/Creativ Collection (NT) (p. 86)
- Goldwell (p. 12 top left, top middle left, top middle right; p. 163)
- Hairtools (p. 56 bottom; p. 122 top and middle; p. 123; p. 124; p. 125; p. 137; p. 158 bottom; p. 160; p. 165 top left and right)
- HSBC (p. 87)
- Haringtons (p. 161; p. 162; p. 163 middle; pp. 168–177; p. 181)
- Ishoka (p. 118; p. 131; p. 147)
- L'Oréal Professional (p. 95)
- Tony Maleedy (p. 12 top right)
- Mark Glenn Hair Enhancement www.markglenn.com (p. 153 middle)
- Oxford Hair Foundation (p. 12 middle)
- George Paterson (p. 49; p. 100; p. 136; p. 157; p. 231)
- Photodisc 75 (NT) (p. 212; p. 213)
- Prestige Medical (p. 56 top)
- Redken Laboratories Ltd (p. 231 top)
- Sally Hair & Beauty (p. 144 bottom; p. 236 bottom)
- Science Photo Library (p. 12 middle left, middle right, bottom left; p. 15 top left, middle left, middle right, bottom left, bottom right)
- Martin Sookias (p. 23; p. 96; p. 97; p. 98; p. 104; p. 128; p. 144 top; p. 149 middle and bottom; p. 150; p. 151; p. 162; p. 187; p. 190; p. 199; p. 207; p. 208; p. 210; p. 225; p. 243; p. 248; p. 256; p. 257; p. 258)
- Sorisa (p. 56 middle)
- Alison Stewart (p. 17; p. 25; p. 51; p. 158 middle; p. 214; p. 232)
- Wahl (p. 133; p. 199)
- Wella (p. 39; p. 40; p. 103; p. 114; p. 115; p. 122; p. 139; p. 146; p. 158, p. 164; p. 180; p. 188; p. 202)
- Wellcome Trust Medical Photographic Library (p. 12 bottom right; p. 15 top right; p. 152; p. 185)
- www.Afrocare.com (p. 153)

Picture research by Eve Thould and Sue Sharp.

The author and publishers acknowledge HABIA as originators and copyright owners of the NVQ occupational standards for hairdressing.

Introduction

Hairdressing is much more than being able to pick up a pair of scissors. You will need to develop lots of different practical skills, such as styling, colouring and perming, to produce an individual hairstyle for your client, making them want to return to you again and again. There is always a reason why everything is done a certain way in hairdressing, such as the way the hairdressing scissors are always held with the thumb and third finger so that you can cut the hair at every angle. This basic knowledge is known as the 'theory side' of hairdressing. Once you understand this knowledge you can explain your techniques to other hairdressers and to your clients, should they ask.

This book explains in simple, practical terms what you will need to know to become a good, competent hairdresser. It starts with client care and works through consultation, hair disorders and diseases, selling skills, stock control, performing well at work, health and safety, reception, shampooing, conditioning and scalp massage, blow drying, setting short and long hair, plaiting and adding hair, cutting and men's barbering techniques, perming, relaxing and neutralising and colouring and bleaching. It is particularly suitable for anyone taking the City & Guilds, SVQ, Edexcel or VTCT Level 2 NVQ (National Vocational Qualification), as it covers all the mandatory and optional units involved.

Always remember that the most important person is the client; salons cannot exist without them! Clients will visit the salon for a variety of reasons.

- They want to *look good* by benefiting from professional hairdressing services, such as:

  cutting, either to create a new style or to reshape the same one;

  perming, to create volume and bounce in the style;

  colouring, to achieve a lighter or brighter colour or to blend in a few grey hairs.
- They want to *feel good* by relaxing in a pleasant atmosphere, feeling that they are in safe hands because the hairdressers are properly trained.

There are several different types of client – regular, occasional or new – but all of them must be treated with respect, courtesy and pleasantness *every* time they enter the salon. Good communication skills are vital – have you ever been put off using a certain shop because the staff were miserable and unhelpful? Therefore, you will need to become an expert hairdresser *and* a good communicator to ensure your clients keep on coming.

Clients today are very well informed from the media (television, radio and magazines) and will often ask about the hairdressing products being used on their hair. You will need a thorough knowledge of hairdressing chemicals and equipment and why some are better than others – especially if they are expensive!

People are attracted to hairdressing salons in a variety of ways, sometimes by advertising or press features, sometimes by word of mouth, but often by the appearance of the salon. A clean, bright and tidy shop with an attractive reception area and smiling, efficient staff often encourages new customers to enter. Remember, the more clients you have the more successful the salon will be.

Salons can be extremely varied and are not only found in the high street. They can also be within:

- large department stores
- cruise liners
- hotels
- health farms
- clinics
- health and fitness clubs
- gymnasiums and leisure centres
- clients' homes (if the hairdresser is freelance)
- hospitals
- prisons
- residential homes
- holiday resorts
- the armed forces
- large businesses.

A career in hairdressing can progress in many different directions – from being a famous hairstylist such as Vidal Sassoon or Nicky Clarke to owning your own salon or working in the film or television world.

Becoming a qualified hairdresser

This means obtaining the City & Guilds, SVQ, Edexcel or VTCT Level 2 NVQ certificate.

There are three major routes to training:

- college training
- private schools
- salon training (Modern Apprenticeships).

More information is available through the Lead Body – Hairdressing and Beauty Industry Authority (HABIA). Look at www.habia.org.uk for information on training in your local area.

Levels of training

There are four levels of training:

- Level 1 – an induction to hairdressing, often taken during school placements. This includes shampooing, conditioning and drying hair, helping with perming, relaxing, colouring and reception, and supporting the hairdressing team, including health and safety matters.
- Level 2 – junior stylist/barber. The knowledge required for this level is covered in this book.
- Level 3 – stylist/senior stylist. The knowledge for this is covered in *Advanced Hairdressing* by Stephanie Henderson and Jan Chivell. This includes client consultation, Indian head massage, fashion cutting, dressing long hair and hair

extentions, specialist colouring, perming and afro hair work, planning and putting on salon shows and promotions and making your salon more profitable.

- Level 4 – management.

Careers in hairdressing

Here are some examples of the many and varied careers available in the hairdressing world.

Film, television and theatrical work

You will need extra qualifications in wig making and make-up, plus some more practical experience with local theatrical companies. There are very few openings: the BBC, for instance, have thousands of applicants for only one or two places. You will also need to be prepared to work all sorts of strange hours when you are needed.

Managerial work

Once you are a qualified stylist you can progress to become a style or artistic director, an educational director, manager or manageress or a salon owner.

Working for a manufacturer

Manufacturers (such as Wella or L'Oréal) employ:

- sales representatives – who sell products to hairdressers
- technical representatives – who give technical advice on products
- demonstrators – who demonstrate hairdressing products in salons, training centres, colleges or within the manufacturers' own schools.

Teaching

Once you are an experienced stylist you can progress to teaching in colleges or training centres, but you will need an advanced qualification such as the City & Guilds, SVQ, Edexcel or VTCT Level III and a recognised teaching qualification. There are the TDLB A and V Assessors Awards for those who wish to assess their trainees.

Trichologist

Hairdressers often refer clients with hair and scalp disorders to a doctor or a trichologist. A trichologist is a hair and scalp specialist who deals with various problems such as hair loss. It takes several years to qualify through the Institute of Trichologists. Once qualified, you can work in either a hair clinic or a hairdressing salon.

It is often said that you never stop learning in hairdressing. You have chosen one of the most interesting, exciting and demanding careers around – enjoy the book and enjoy your hairdressing career!

Portfolios

What is a portfolio?

Your portfolio is a collection of both the work that you can do now (e.g. photographs of the blow drys you have done) and of work that you may have done in the past (e.g. a diploma from a manufacturer's hair colouring school). The intention is to show that you can do your job well.

This work that you collect is called evidence, and is a necessary part of gaining your qualification and certificates.

You will normally need a large ring-binder file to keep all your (A4) sheets of evidence. Paper sheets are best kept in clear plastic envelopes with small sticky labels (for numbering and indexing later) stuck to the top outside corners.

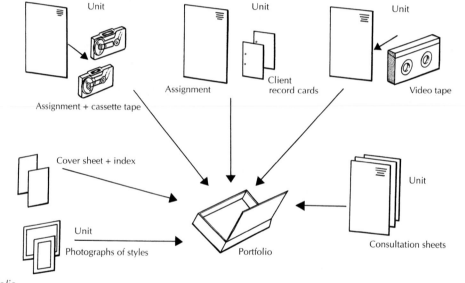

Portfolio

A box file may also be useful for keeping any video or cassette tapes or other pieces of evidence.

Section cards in your file are particularly useful to keep each area, such as your personal information, index system and each unit of work, separate.

What should your portfolio contain?

A cover sheet

This should give details of your centre (name, address and telephone number), the qualification (e.g. NVQ Level 2 Hairdressing) you are working for and your name (and candidate number, if known).

BASIC HAIRDRESSING

Personal information

Only include what is relevant to the award (your certificate), e.g. your job description if you are working in a salon or a personal account of your work history (you may have experienced working with the public within paid or voluntary work).

People involved in the assessment

You should include the names of people who train, assess or verify your work.

Assessment record book

This may be kept inside your portfolio or held separately. The table below gives a brief description of some of the terms often used.

Terms often used in a portfolio

TITLE	DESCRIPTION
Candidate	Someone registered with C&G/Edexcel or VTCT to take the certificate
Assessor	A qualified person who decides if your work is of the required standard then ticks, signs and dates with you when you have completed the work
Internal verifier	A qualified person who checks the assessment record books, the portfolios and the assessor's judgement of your practical work
External verifier	A qualified person who comes to your centre to check up on all the work
ARB	Assessment record book
Unit	An area or subject, e.g. cutting, reception
Outcome	A smaller part of a unit
Mandatory unit	A unit you have to do
Optional unit	A unit you choose to do
Additional unit	An extra unit that you do by choice
Performance criteria	These state what you must do to perform a relevant task – for example, how to shampoo correctly
Range statements	These specify the contexts or variables that must be covered, e.g. how to shampoo dry, normal, greasy and dandruff-affected hair
Essential knowledge and understanding	This is the background information that you need to know, and is contained within this book

A unit checklist

This is often provided by your centre and is completed as soon as you finish each unit, to check your progress. Remember, you can gain accreditation in one or more units if that is what you wish.

An individual action plan

This is provided by your centre to help you to know how much and what evidence you will need to provide for each unit and if you will need any further training.

An index

This is a description of how you have organised your work, for example:

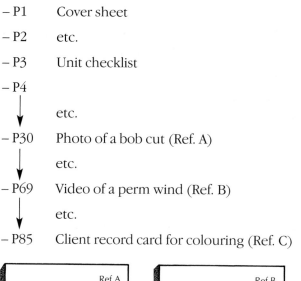

- P1   Cover sheet
- P2   etc.
- P3   Unit checklist
- P4
        etc.
- P30   Photo of a bob cut (Ref. A)
        etc.
- P69   Video of a perm wind (Ref. B)
        etc.
- P85   Client record card for colouring (Ref. C)

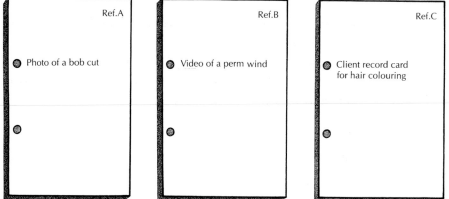

| Ref.A | Ref.B | Ref.C |
| Photo of a bob cut | Video of a perm wind | Client record card for hair colouring |

Examples of portfolio index

Unit evidence

The unit evidence will contain:

- records of observation by your assessor (e.g. someone has watched and recorded you shampooing)
- records of any oral questions asked by your assessor (these may be recorded on cassette tape)
- products of your performance, e.g.
  - photographs or videos of hairstyles you have produced (try to include yourself in the photo)
  - client record cards
  - consultation sheets or reports about your work
  - memos (recording that you have taken telephone messages correctly)
  - any other relevant information such as letters, drawings or computer printouts
- evidence from other people, such as letters or reports from managers, other members of staff, clients or other observers (these are called witness testimonies)
- certificates, e.g. colouring or perming diplomas from manufacturers' schools

- supplementary evidence, such as projects, assignments, simulations, case studies or records of oral questions that cover any gaps in your evidence. This will ensure that you have covered the range (all the work).

All your evidence must be:
- valid – it must relate to the standards (what is written in your assessment book)
- authentic – it must be what you have done, and no one else
- current – it must show that you can currently do the work
- sufficient – there must be enough evidence to prove that you have covered all the work in your assessment book.

Do's and don'ts

Do:
- ask your trainer or assessor if you need help
- constantly look at your assessment book to check the requirements
- ask others to help provide witness testimonies
- use illustrations or photographs
- cross-reference wherever you can, e.g. use the same set of photographs for cutting, perming and conditioning
- explain things clearly, using simple terms and step-by-step techniques
- present your portfolio in a professional manner – it must be legible and readers should easily be able find what they are looking for.

Don't:
- make your work any longer than it needs to be
- leave any areas uncompleted
- accidently retain your written assessments – they should be kept by your assessors in a locked file (to be checked by the External Verifier)
- lose or mislay any work – you might have to do it all again!
- keep your formative assessments (which is when you have done the work but it is not yet up to the required standard) in your portfolio.

REMEMBER

All of your summative assessments (which show that the work you have produced is of the required standard) must be in your portfolio.

Unit / Chapters	G1	G4	G5	G6	G7	G8	H2	H6	H8	H9	H10	H11	H12	H13	H14	H15	H16	H17	H18
1. Client communications			✓	✓	✓														
2. Performing well at work						✓													
3. Health, safety and security in the salon	✓																		
4. Reception		✓																	
5. Shampoo and conditioning										✓									✓
6. Blow drying, setting and dressing											✓	✓							
7. Cutting								✓											
8. Men's haircutting							✓		✓									✓	
9. Perming, relaxing and neutralising													✓			✓	✓		
10. Colouring and bleaching														✓					

Chapter 1 Client communications

After working through this chapter you will be able to:

- Understand your own responsibilities under legislation and salon policy
- Create a comfortable atmosphere between you and your client
- Decide how and when to carry out hair and skin tests
- Identify what clients want by using different sources of information
- Analyse the hair, skin and scalp
- Advise your client and agree services and products
- Understand who your clients are and what they want
- Know how to give your clients what they want and bring them back into the salon
- Understand all the products and services offered by your salon
- Identify which products and services the client needs
- Deliver information using good communication techniques
- Gain client commitment to using additional products or services.

This chapter covers the following NVQ Level 2 units:
Advise and Consult with Clients
Give Clients a Positive Impression of Yourself and Your Organisation
Promote Additional Services and Products to Clients

Introduction

Client consultation means talking to your client and giving advice before starting work on their **hair**.
During this consultation you will also be examining your client's hair by brushing it through. In the same way that doctors diagnose their patients' illnesses, you will be able to diagnose any hair or **scalp** conditions and take the appropriate action.

REMEMBER

Clients may have no idea of what they want. This is your opportunity to make recommendations and to build up a good relationship, which may lead to a return visit.

HEALTH MATTERS

Standing all day long

Shoulders
Work with your shoulders relaxed. Exercise helps by contracting and relaxing the muscles. Try raising your shoulders by lifting them up towards your ears and letting them drop. It is possible to do six of these in ten seconds, so try to do it at least twice a day.

You will also be able to assess the client's requirements generally, and make recommendations for a **hairstyle** to suit their appearance and lifestyle..

Gaining information

You must find out:
* the client's name
* the service (e.g. cut, perm, colour) required
* the chosen hairstyle (you may need to use a style book).

Record keeping

Why bother to keep client records?

* Another stylist will be able to attend to a client when the normal stylist is away (off sick or on holiday).
* It is possible to check when the client last visited your salon for a colour or a perm (some salons send out reminder cards).
* The **clientele** feel they are being professionally treated when they see you are checking their personal records.
* You are able to know exactly what perm lotion at which strength and what **curler** size was used on previous occasions (especially useful if the perm was too tight or too soft last time).
* You are able to know what make of colour or bleach was used on previous occasions, which colour was used, the peroxide strength and the length of time the hair took to process.
* Any conditioning treatments recorded will allow you to know how many were needed before the hair returned to good condition.
* You can keep details of any special conditions, such as any medication the client has been taking, or details of a **resistant section of hair**.
* You can deal with any complaints more efficiently. For example, if a client complains that a perm has not lasted, but your records show that the perm used was a very soft perm which was only intended to last six to eight weeks, you can remind the client of those details.
* You will have a record of the client's telephone number and address, which may be needed if an appointment has to be changed.

Records are generally kept for perming, **hair colouring** and bleaching, and for conditioning treatments.

Record cards

Record cards are stored either in a filing box or in a filing cabinet, in alphabetical order according to the surnames of the clients.

Cards must be filled in and filed back in alphabetical order after use.

Some salons design their own record cards; others buy or use specially made cards.

Client name							Special notes	
Address								
							Homecare sales	
Daytime telephone no.								
Date	Stylist	Scalp condition	Hair condition	Technique	Products	Develop-ment time	Result	

Example record card

Computers

Many salons now use computers, not only for recording all the takings but also for keeping client records. You will have to be trained to use such computers properly. All computers are operated by a program, which is known as the software. Salon computer software will need to classify, store and retrieve information: the type of software used to do this is known as a database.

Once all the client records are on the database, then retrieving the information is quick and easy.

Client consultation

TO DO
- *Watch and note how the stylists in your salon perform a consultation.*
- *Practise talking politely to clients about their hair.*
- *Practise making a mental note of the height, size, face shape, age, personality, lifestyle and occupation of your clients.*

Experienced hairdressers will be able to produce a perfect hairstyle for each individual client by considering:

- **face shape** (oval, round, long or square)
- approximate height (tall or short)
- approximate size (thin or overweight)
- approximate age (not everyone can take 'young' styles)
- skin colour
- lifestyle (busy people want a hairstyle that is quick and easy to manage)
- personality (quiet and shy or lively and outgoing)
- occupation (some professions may have strict rules about hair length)
- cost (make sure a price list is accessible)
- medical history (some illnesses affect perming and tinting)
- occasion (dinner dance, wedding)
- time available (can the client spare the time for a long process such as perming?).

NB: All this should be done before gowning up the client so that you can consider their clothes and lifestyle, and see their height and body shape more clearly.

REMEMBER
All consultations are done on dry hair before shampooing. You cannot always see the problems (e.g. dry ends) when the hair is wet.

REMEMBER
Allow enough time to complete your consultation checklist and always check it with your supervisor.

Talking to clients

Your communication skills are just as important when working with new clients as they are with regular clients. Smiling at others encourages good humour and a pleasant manner. It is very difficult not to smile back at someone who smiles at you.

- Look at your client in the mirror or face to face. Eye contact can express friendliness and trust, showing that you are paying attention.
- Listen to your client. Many clients never return to a salon because, although they have been given a lovely new hairstyle, it was not the one they asked for!
- Speak to your client and explain any reasons for delays straight away, and in a tactful manner. Always be honest and factual. If the client is rushed for time or appears rather cross then ask your supervisor to help.

Remember that a satisfied client is good for business. A happy client will tell a few people about you, while an unhappy client tells everyone. Clients have every right to expect the service they agreed to have and have paid for.

By giving advice to clients you are promoting the salon and yourself as a technical expert. It is also the best way of 'selling' to a client.

Handling difficult clients

- Be courteous, friendly, calm and understanding.
- Do not pass judgement or argue.
- Do listen, offer understanding and help clarify the problem.
- Give technical explanations.
- Ensure you have good body language and maintain good eye contact.
- Make sure communications are clear.

Always inform a senior staff member if the client is unhappy, as they can often help remedy the matter and resolve the problem.

Complaints that are dealt with quickly and with good customer service will mean that the client is more likely to continue to visit the salon.

Confused clients

These clients require clear and precise clarification to enable them to understand. It is important to ensure that you understand what it is the client is confused about to enable you to clarify any uncertainties.

TEST YOUR KNOWLEDGE

1 Describe why it is important to communicate effectively with your client.
2 All client consultation checklists and record cards are confidential. Why is this important?
3 How do the requirements of the Data Protection Act affect you?
4 Describe how verbal communication should be conducted.

Gowning up

Ideally the stylist will always carry out a consultation with the client before gowning up, so that the client's clothes and lifestyle, height and build can be observed beforehand. Always check with the stylist when they would like you to gown up a client.

Gowning up is necessary to protect:
- the client's clothes from becoming wet, from falling hair clippings, perm lotion, colours and bleaches
- the client's eyes and skin during chemical processes such as perming, **neutralising**, relaxing, colouring and bleaching (see 'Cotton wool strips' below).

Gowns

Gowns should always be freshly laundered and tied securely. Some salons use different coloured gowns for different purposes – for example darker gowns (sometimes plastic) for colouring, perming or bleaching.

Towels

Clean towels should be used for every client and must be placed securely around the client's neck. They are to be used within the salon during shampooing and chemical processes. Some salons use two towels: one around the front and one around the back; while others secure the ends of one towel with a butterfly clamp. Again, check the colour of towel to be used – darker ones are often used for colouring.

Cotton wool strips

Many salons use these to protect the client during perming and neutralising so that the lotion does not run on to the client's skin or into their eyes. The strip is usually dampened with water before being applied so that the perm lotion or neutraliser is not absorbed into the cotton wool strip from the hair.

Neck strips

Neck strips are placed between the towel or gown and the client's neck to prevent any hair clippings or chemicals falling on the client's clothes.

Barrier cream

This is carefully applied around the client's **hairline** (not on the hair) to prevent skin being stained by colours or to protect sensitive skin during bleaching or relaxing. Sometimes barrier cream is placed on the scalp as an extra protection during chemical relaxing.

Cutting collars

These are usually placed around the shoulders during cutting so that the hair falls easily from the collar.

REMEMBER

Your client is paying for a service, so always be professional, polite and helpful.
Make sure that the client is kept safe in the salon.
Make sure the client is fully protected by gowning properly and that belongings are kept with the client at all times.

TO DO

Watch your supervisor gowning up a client in preparation for:
- shampooing
- cutting
- perming
- hair colouring
- bleaching.

REMEMBER

Always offer the client refreshments and/or reading materials as part of your service.

REMEMBER

Always check that the client has removed large earrings, other jewellery (e.g. necklaces) or glasses if necessary before gowning up. Ask the client to keep them in a safe place (in a bag for instance).
Make sure you tuck the client's clothing inside the gown, especially high-necked jumpers.

Examining the hair and scalp

Finding out what the client wants to have done to their hair and choosing a style is very important, but sometimes the hairdressing service that is possible depends entirely on what the client's hair and scalp condition will allow.

For instance, if the hair is untreated it means that no chemicals have been used on it, but if it has been chemically treated it will react differently to **blow drying** and **setting**, **perming**, colouring and **bleaching**.

A temporary colour (a coloured **mousse** or setting lotion) affects different parts of the hair than a permanent colour (a tint) does. You will need to recognise the different parts of the hair and learn how they are affected by various chemicals, and whether coloured hair can be permed, coloured or bleached in future.

Hair can be damaged by chemical treatments. It can also be damaged by handling – bad brushing, excessive blow drying or tonging. Again, you will need to know what part of the hair is damaged and whether further services can be carried out.

As you are carrying out your consultation you can start to diagnose your client's hair condition. In order to understand why some people have shiny, manageable hair in good condition, while others have very difficult hair, you need to know more about hair structure.

Hair structure

Each hair is made up of three layers – in a similar way to a pencil.

- The outside layer, the **cuticle**, is thin and flat (like the paint on the outside of a pencil).
- The middle layer, the **cortex**, is the strong, main part of the hair (like the wood of the pencil).
- The central layer, the **medulla**, runs finely through the middle (like the lead in a pencil).

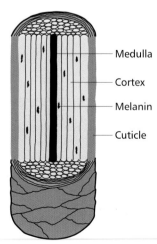

Medulla

Cortex

Melanin

Cuticle

Longitudinal section through a hair

The cuticle

If you look carefully at the diagrams you will see that the cuticle is actually made up of overlapping scales (7–10 layers). These scales look like the tiles on a roof, with the edges of the scales all lying away from the scalp. They are **translucent**, like frosted glass, so that the hair colour (in the cortex) can be seen through them.

This outside layer of the **hair shaft** is very tough and holds the whole hair together, but it may be damaged by strong chemicals (such as perms or bleaches) or harsh treatments (such as too much **back-brushing**).

Once the cuticle scales have been damaged or broken and have opened up, and chemicals have been absorbed into the cortex, the hair surface will look and feel rough and dull (like sandpaper). If the scales are undamaged and closed tight and flat, then the hair will appear beautifully shiny (like glass).

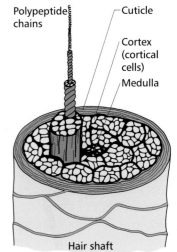

Cross-section through a hair

The cortex

The cortex is the main part of the hair, lying underneath the cuticle. Hairdressers need to understand the cortex because this is where all the changes take place when the hair is blow-dried, **set**, permed, tinted and bleached.

It is made from many strands or fibres, which are twisted together like knitting wool. These can stretch, then return to their original length.

Hair is made of a protein called **keratin**, itself made up from amino acid units, which are found in long coiled chains called **polypeptide chains**. All the coils of polypeptide chains are held together by various links and bonds.

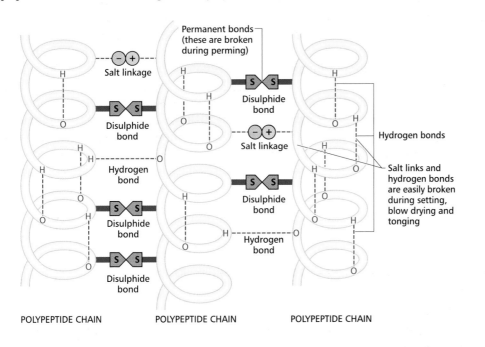

The structure of keratin

Look at the diagram and find the temporary bonds. These are the hydrogen bonds and **salt links**. They break and rejoin wherever hair is blow-dried, set, tonged or hot brushed into a different style. They are called temporary bonds because all of these processes are easily reversed by dampening the hair and starting again.

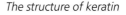

There are also permanent bonds in the diagram: these are called **disulphide bonds**. Disulphide bonds are very strong and can be broken only by using a strong chemical such as permanent **wave** lotion on the hair.

The cortex also contains all the colour pigments in the hair. These pigments are called **melanin** (brown/black) and **pheomelanin** (yellow/red).

The medulla

The medulla does not have any real function. It is not always present in scalp hairs, particularly if the hair is fine.

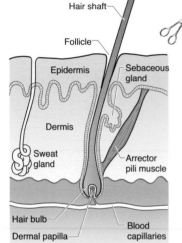

The structure of the skin

Scalp (or skin) structure

There are two main types of hair on the human body. Fine **vellus hair** grows on the body and stronger **terminal hair** grows on the scalp (and makes up eyebrows, eyelashes, beards and moustaches). A third type of hair, **lanugo hair**, is only found on human fetuses and is even finer than vellus hair. The scalp is stronger than the rest of the body skin (which is why we can put chemicals on scalp hair without causing too much damage), but its structure is otherwise similar to body skin.

Hair is made of the protein keratin, which is dead. There are no nerve endings inside hair and so it does not hurt when we cut through it, or when chemicals such as perm lotions or bleaches are put on to it.

However, we can feel someone pulling our hair because it is attached to the scalp by its root, sitting in a tiny pocket called the hair **follicle**. Nerve endings attached to the hair root tell us when our hair is being pulled and when a hair should stand on end. We all have occasional 'goose pimples', the hair standing on end if we are very cold or frightened. The **arrector pili muscle** is attached to the hair root and contracts (or squeezes together) to pull the hair upright, creating the goose pimples.

The **sebaceous gland** is also attached to the hair follicle and produces **sebum**, the hair's natural oil or lubricant. The sebum flows around the hair root and outwards on to the scalp surface. If too much sebum is produced the scalp and hair are too greasy, but if too little sebum is produced the hair and scalp are too dry.

The scalp (and skin) is divided into two layers:
- the outer layer – the **epidermis** – is the outer protective layer of skin. It is constantly shedding itself, losing dead skin cells. When this happens excessively on the scalp it is known as **dandruff**
- the inner layer – the **dermis** – is the thickest and most important part of the skin. It is where the hair follicles, nerve endings, sebaceous glands, blood supply and sweat glands are found.

Hair could not grow without its own blood supply. The heart pumps blood containing food and oxygen (needed to make new keratin) through the arteries towards the skin surface. The arteries become small **blood capillaries** in the dermis, where they feed blood into the bottom of the hair root or follicle to feed the **dermal papilla**. The more blood there is flowing towards the **hair papilla** the more the hair will grow. Therefore, when our skins are red and warm in the summer, our hair (and nails) grow more quickly.

We can also regulate the body temperature through the skin through **sweat glands**. These produce sweat, which flows on to the skin through the pores, cooling the body down when it evaporates.

TO DO

- *Copy the diagram of the skin structure and then try to label it up on your own.*
- *Describe the structure of the scalp or skin in your own words.*

Hair growth and life cycle

Hair grows from the bottom of its root at the dermal papilla, where new cells are constantly being produced. These soft cells become hardened to form strong hair above the skin surface. The average rate of hair growth is 1.25 cm ($\frac{1}{2}$ in) per month. This amount of hair growth keeps hairdressers in business!

There are approximately 100,000 hairs growing on the average scalp, and there is a constant daily loss of 50–100 scalp hairs. We lose these hairs because every so often the hair follicle has a period of rest, and so the hair falls out.

The **hair growth cycle** has three stages. The growing stage of the hair is called the **anagen** stage. When the hair starts to go into its resting state, it is said to be in the **catagen** stage. The resting stage is called the **telogen** stage.

Obviously not all hairs rest at the same time – or we would go bald!

TO DO

Look again at the typical growth rate of hair. Work out how often you should recommend your client to return for:
- *cutting*
- *perming*
- *highlights*
- *permanent hair colouring.*

REMEMBER

The word ACT:
    A = Anagen
    C = Catagen
    T = Telogen.

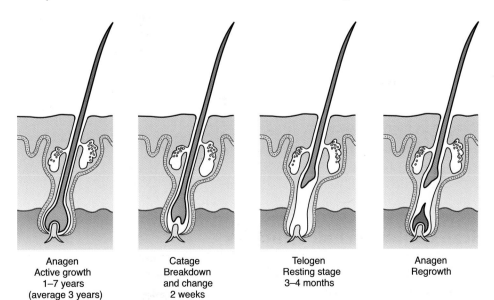

Anagen	Catage	Telogen	Anagen
Active growth	Breakdown	Resting stage	Regrowth
1–7 years	and change	3–4 months	
(average 3 years)	2 weeks		

Hair growth life cycle

The diagram shows how the hair gradually stops growing and starts again.

TEST YOUR KNOWLEDGE

1 Describe a typical growth speed for hair.
2 Copy the hair growth life cycle diagram and try to label it without looking in your book.
3 Explain in your own words why hairdressers need to know about hair growth life cycles.

Each hair grows for between $1\frac{1}{2}$ and seven years before reaching a resting stage. This means that some clients' hair will grow to shoulder length:

$$1\frac{1}{2} \text{ years} \times 1.25 \text{ cm } (\tfrac{1}{2}\text{ in}) \text{ per month} = 22.5 \text{ cm } (9 \text{ in})$$

but other clients' hair will grow down to their waist or longer:

$$7 \text{ years} \times 1.25 \text{ cm } (\tfrac{1}{2}\text{ in}) \text{ per month} = 105 \text{ cm } (42 \text{ inches}).$$

So when a client complains that they cannot grow long hair you can explain to them that it is because their hair has a short life cycle.

Hair shape

There are three basic hair shapes: straight, wavy and curly.

The shape of the hair is created in the hair follicle at the anagen stage. As the hair is pushed up through the follicle, it takes on the shape and curve of the follicle.

A cross-section of a hair shows that hair with:

- a round diameter usually produces straight hair
- an oval diameter usually produces wavy hair
- a kidney-shaped or flattened diameter usually produces **curly hair**.

Cell growth in the papilla also plays an important part of hair shaping; if the cell growth is greater on one side than on the other, it creates an uneven shape, the hair bends naturally to the shorter side, creating natural curl.

Ethnic structural hair types

There are three main racial differences in hair types:

- **European hair – Caucasian** – is generally wavy
- Asian hair – **Mongoloid** – is usually straight
- **African Caribbean** hair – is usually curly.

Each type of hair will react differently to different hairdressing processes.

African Caribbean hair structure

African Caribbean hair is naturally dark because it contains more melanin. It also needs more care and conditioning than Caucasian (European) hair because of its curly and crinkly shape. It tends to tangle easily, and may be damaged and break at the ends simply by being **disentangled** with **combs** and brushes.

Straight hair

Hair follicle

Epidermis

Dermal papilla

Wavy hair

Curly hair

Hair shapes

Its curl is formed because of uneven keratinisation. This means that the keratin in the hair is more dense on the inside of the curl or wave – the 'para' cortex – and less dense on the outside of the curl or wave – the 'ortho' cortex.

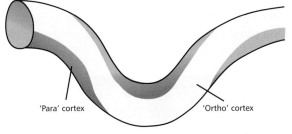

'Para' cortex   'Ortho' cortex

Afro hair structure

African Caribbean hair has slightly more cuticle layers than Caucasian hair and is therefore initially more resistant to chemical processes such as tinting, bleaching, perming and relaxing. Because it has more cuticle it has less volume of cortex, and once chemicals have entered through the cuticle and into the cortex they will process African Caribbean hair more quickly than Caucasian hair.

Hair thickness

This is known as hair **texture**, and is determined by the thickness of each individual hair – whether it is coarse, medium or fine.

Very fine hair

TO DO

- Pull out three hairs from your head: one from the front, the middle and the back.
- Ask several friends to do the same.
- Compare the thickness of each individual hair against a sheet of paper.

Density

Average hair

Density is measured by the amount of hairs per square centimetre (cm²) on the scalp. Hair density is described as follows.

- Sparse/thin: few hairs per cm². Looking down the hair mesh more scalp than hair is seen.
- Medium: the ratio of hair to scalp per cm² is equal.
- Dense/thick/abundant: lots of hair per cm². Looking down the hair mesh, more hair than scalp is seen.

The width of the hair sections that should be taken when winding and during the application of treatments and tints is determined by hair density.

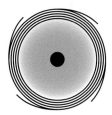

Very coarse hair

Hair thickness

- Dense/thick hair needs small/fine sections per **rod**, to prevent a weak curl or patchy application finish.
- Sparse/thin hair can have larger sections. Pulling the hair towards the roller or rod must be prevented, as this can cause distorted hair shapes, or even break the hair.

Hair and scalp conditions

These may be:
- non-infectious – they cannot be spread from one client to another, for example **alopecia (baldness)**

REMEMBER

Some people have very **fine hair**, but lots and lots of it, while some people have very coarse hair but not very much of it.

- infectious – they can be spread from one client to another, for example **head lice**.

Non-infectious hair and scalp conditions

Although a non-infectious or non-**contagious** disorder may appear unsightly, it cannot be spread from one person to another and can be treated in the salon.

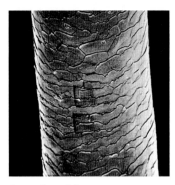

Smooth cuticles

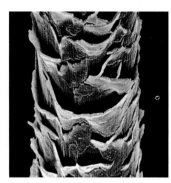

Damaged cuticles

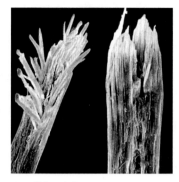

Fragilitis crinium

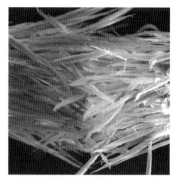

Trichorrhexis nodosa

Monilethrix

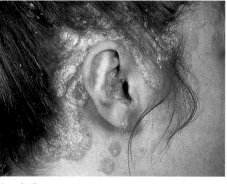

Psoriasis

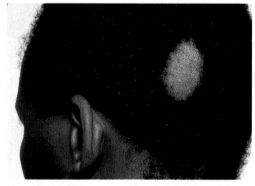

Alopecia areata

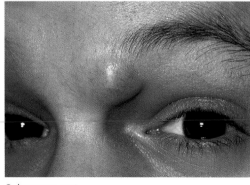

Sebaceous cyst

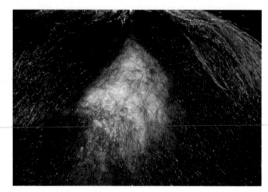

Cicatrical alopecia

NAME	DESCRIPTION	CAUSE	TREATMENT
Pityriasis capitis (dandruff)	Small, itchy, dry scales, white or grey coloured	Overactive production and shedding of epidermal cells Stress related	Anti-dandruff **shampoos** Oil **conditioners** or conditioning creams applied to the scalp
Seborrhoea (greasiness)	Excessive oil on the scalp or skin	Overactive sebaceous gland	Shampoos for greasy hair Spirit lotions
Eczema	Red, inflamed skin which can develop into splitting and weeping areas. It is often irritated, sore and painful	Either a physical irritation or an allergic reaction	Medical treatment
Fragilitis crinium (**split ends**)	Split, dry, roughened hair ends	Harsh physical or chemical damage	Cutting and reconditioning treatments
Damaged cuticle (tangled hair)	Cuticle scales roughened and damaged, hair dull	Harsh physical or chemical damage	Reconditioning treatments Restructurants
Trichorrhexis nodosa (swollen, broken hair shaft)	Hair roughened and swollen along the hair shaft, sometimes broken off	Harsh use of chemicals (e.g. perm rubbers fastened too tightly during perming) Physical damage (e.g. from elastic bands)	Restructurants Recondition and cut hair where possible
Monilethrix (beaded hair shaft)	Beaded hair (a very rare condition)	Uneven production of keratin in the follicle	Treat this hair very gently within the salon
Psoriasis (silver scaling patches)	Thick, raised, dry, silvery scales often found behind the ears	Overactive production and shedding of the epidermal cells. Possibly passed on in families, recurring in times of stress	Medical treatment and seek medical approval Careful use of tools (especially cutting) Coal tar shampoo
Alopecia areata (round bald patches)	Bald patches, which can be found both on the scalp and on mens's facial hair	Shock or stress Hereditary	Medical treatment and seek medical approval High-frequency treatment Avoid undue hair **tension**
Male-pattern baldness (baldness, thinning hair)	Receding hairline, thinning hair	Genetic or hereditary baldness	Medical treatment is being developed
Cicatrical (scarring) alopecia	A permanent bald patch where the hair follicles have been destroyed	A scar from skin damage caused by chemicals, heat or a cut	None
Sebaceous cyst (lump on scalp)	A lump either on top of or just underneath the scalp	Blockage of the sebaceous gland	Medical treatment Careful use of tools
Moles	Usually a small harmless raised or flat area. May be pigmented or not, smooth or rough, hairy or hairless	Pigmented moles are caused by an overgrowth of melanocytes (cells that produce hair and skin colour = melanin). Changes to the shape or size of moles should be referred to a medical practitioner	Careful use of tools Changes to the shape and size of the mole should be referred to a medical practitioner It is safe to cut the hairs from hairy moles but not to pluck them, which disturbs the skin cells

For illustrations of non-infectious **diseases**, see the colour photographs on page 12.

Infectious hair and scalp conditions

Infestations or infectious disorders must not be treated in the salon.
Deal with the client sympathetically and tactfully. Explain that you have found a certain hair or scalp condition, which means that you cannot continue with their hair service. You must then recommend that the client seeks medical advice from either a doctor or a **trichologist** (a specialist in hair and scalp disorders).

All equipment must be cleaned and **sterilised** after contact with such a condition (see Chapter 3).

For illustrations of infectious diseases, see the colour photographs on pages 15.

Infectious diseases and conditions of the hair and scalp

DISEASE	DESCRIPTION	CAUSE
Infestations		
Pediculosis capitis (head lice)	Highly infectious Small, grey **parasites** with six legs, 2 mm ($\frac{1}{12}$ in) long, which bite the scalp and suck blood. The female insects lay eggs called 'nits', which are cemented to the hair Very common in children	Infestation of head lice, which lay eggs, producing more lice living off human blood Treatment is by combing with a fine tooth comb over well-conditioned hair or using special shampoos or lotions
Scabies	An itchy rash found in the folds of the the skin. Reddish spots and burrows (greyish lines) under the skin	A tiny animal mite which burrows through skin to lay its eggs
Infections		
Tinea capitis (ringworm)	Highly infectious Pink patches on the scalp develop into round, grey scaly areas with broken hairs It is most common in children	**Fungus** spread indirectly through brushes, combs or by direct contact (touching) or towels
Impetigo (oozing pustules)	Highly infectious Blisters on the skin which 'weep' then dry to form a yellow crust	**Bacteria** entering through broken or cut skin
Folliculitis (small yellow pustules with hair in centre)	Small yellow pustules with hair in centre	Bacteria from scratching or contact with an infected person

TEST YOUR KNOWLEDGE

1 Starting on the outside, name the three layers of the hair shaft.
2 Describe each infestation, infectious and non-infectious condition and its cause, without looking at your book.
3 List which hair and scalp conditions can be treated in the salon.
4 Describe the treatments that are available for the conditions that can be treated in the salon.

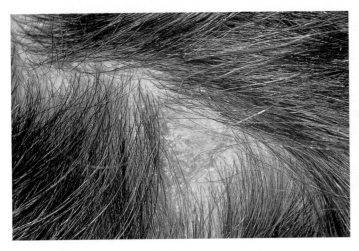

Tinea capitis

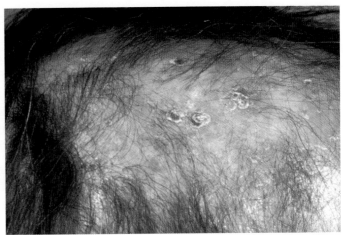

Folliculitis

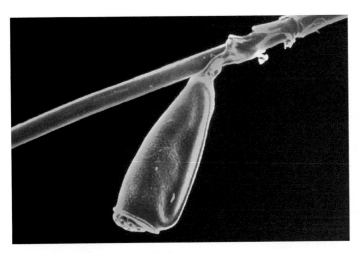

Pediculosis capitis (eggs or 'nits')

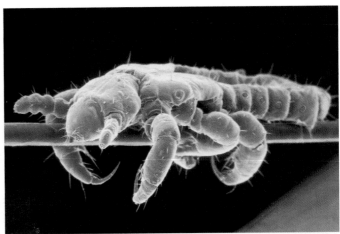

Pediculosis capitis (head louse)

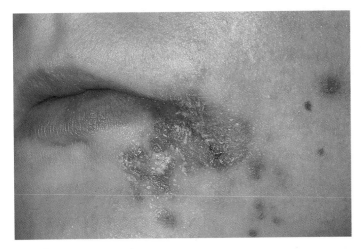

Impetigo

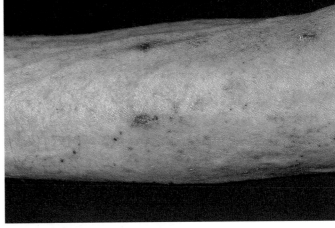

Scabies

Establishing hair condition

Hair in good condition will shine and look great. Clients with a new haircut and hair in good condition will also find that perms, colours and highlights take equally well.

However, hair that is damaged and dry may need special perm lotions or different types of colourants to improve its condition.

Internal and external hair condition

LOCATION	GOOD CONDITION	POOR CONDITION
Surface condition	Cuticle scales lie flat and close together Surface is smooth and shiny	Cuticle scales are raised and open, sometimes damaged Surface is rough and dull, e.g. **fragilitis crinium** (split ends) Damaged cuticle This is known as **porous** hair
Internal condition	The chemical links and bonds in keratin within the cortex are strong and elastic and contain natural moisture	The chemical links and bonds in keratin within the cortex have been broken by strong chemicals, e.g. perm lotion, hydrogen peroxide. This hair has lost strength, elasticity and moisture (through the open cuticle scales). It is known as over-elastic hair (stretchy hair)

REMEMBER

Physical or handling damage is caused by bad brushing and combing (over **back-combing**) or excessive drying (hairdryer too hot, excessive tonging or hot brushing).

Weather damage is caused by excessive exposure to the sun, sea and wind.

Chemical damage is caused by excessive perming, bleaching (highlighting) and tinting.

TEST YOUR KNOWLEDGE

1 List the indicators of hair in good condition.
2 List the indicators of hair in bad condition.

Physical and handling damage

Here are some causes of physical and handling damage:

- bad brushing – disentangling from the roots instead of starting at the ends
- bad combing – over back-combing
- over-drying – the hairdryer too hot and held too close to the hair
- excessive use of electrical appliances – tongs and hot brushes
- excessive tension – especially from rubber bands
- strong sunlight, sea and chlorinated water – hair lightens and dries out
- very windy conditions – cause hair to tangle.

Chemical damage

You already know what chemically **damaged hair** looks like but you need to know some of the reasons why the damage may have happened. For instance, a perm could look straight either because it was **over-processed** (a straight frizz) or because it was **under-processed**. The under-processed perm could possibly be repermed, but the hair of an over-processed perm would be sure to disintegrate and break off if further perming was attempted.

The general reasons why hair may be chemically damaged are:

● clients have used products from the chemist without any professional skill or knowledge
● their previous hairdresser has not carried out a proper consultation or analysed the hair thoroughly
● the hairdresser has misinterpreted the client's requirements
● the hairdresser did not have enough practical skill, product or technical knowledge
● the product was applied badly, left on too long (over-processed) or not long enough (under-processed).

Some specific reasons for chemical damage are:

● perming – hair looks frizzy and may break off (the scalp may be sore or burned)
● **relaxing** – curly hair has been permanently straightened and is starting to break off
● bleaching and highlighting – hair looks and feels 'straw like' and the colour may be patchy
● **tinting** (tint applied on top of tint) – the hair feels very dry and the colour is patchy and uneven
● **colour strippers** – hair may be patchy in colour if strippers are not applied quickly and evenly.

REMEMBER

Always display tact when dealing with incorrectly treated hair. Everyone makes the odd mistake, so be positive and helpful towards your client.

TEST YOUR KNOWLEDGE

State the effects of incorrect application of:

1 bleaches
2 tints
3 perm lotion
4 neutralisers
5 colour strippers.

TO DO

Collect as many cuttings of hair in good and poor condition as you can find in your salon. Stick them down on paper and caption each with possible reasons for the condition.

Designing a hairstyle to suit your client

Have you ever wondered why two clients with exactly the same colour, texture and length of hair and the same hairstyle look quite different? It is not only because of their height and build but also because of their head, face or neck shape. Clients must be advised according to these limitations.

Head shape

The shape of a person's head can be seen clearly when the hair is wet and combed flat against the scalp. If the head is flat on the **crown** for instance, you can compensate for this by leaving the hair longer in that area during cutting.

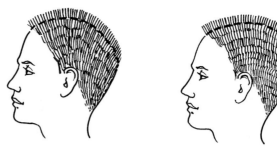

Head shapes for a 'flat top' hairstyle

Head shapes can also look quite different from the front just by altering the parting from side to centre. A side parting will make the head appear broader and wider; a centre parting will make the head appear narrower and thinner.

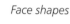
Face shapes

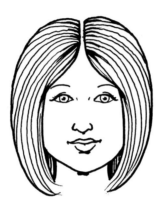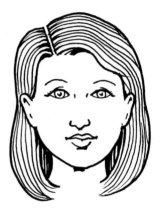

Side and centre parting

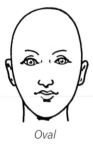
Oval

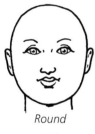
Round

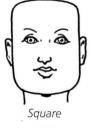
Square

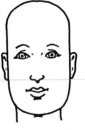
Oblong

Face shapes

There are four main face shapes: oval, round, square and oblong (long).

Oval
An oval face shape is ideal and suits any hairstyle.

Round
Round faces need height to reduce the width of the face. A straight centre parting will also help to reduce the width.

Square
Square-shaped faces need round shapes with wisps of hair on the face to soften them and give the illusion of being oval.

Oblong
Long faces suit short, wider hairstyles dressed around the sides of the face. A low side parting will also make the face look wider.

TO DO
- Comb all your hair away from your face when it is wet and try to decide on your own face shape.
- Make notes on your consultation sheets of different clients' face shapes.
- Check with your supervisor to see if these are correct.

Neck shapes

Long and thin necks are more apparent with short hairstyles, and so need longer hair around them. Short necks can be made to look longer by an unswept or flicked style.

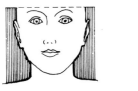 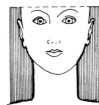 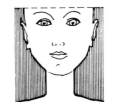

Neck shapes

Ear shapes and levels

Generally, large ears, or even large lobes, are highlighted by a **hair cut** that is short or dressed away from the face. It is better to leave the hair longer over the ears.

Some clients have ears that are uneven, so *never* balance a haircut by the level of the ears.

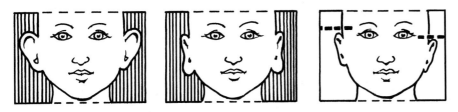

Ear shapes and levels

Nose shapes

A large nose will be more obvious from the side view when hair is drawn back from the face, whereas **dressing** the hair forward helps to minimise it.

Body build and height

One of the main reasons for consultation with the client before gowning up is so that you can briefly judge their body build and height.

Smaller clients can look overwhelmed by too much hair or can be made to appear shorter from the back by wearing their hair too long.

On the other hand, large or overweight clients need a style with some **volume** and length to create a balance between their heads and their bodies. Short, flat hairstyles can highlight large bodies.

Age

A client's age is always an important consideration. Sometimes it is difficult to judge how old a person is, but generally softer styles with more movement are flattering on older people. Avoid straight angular shapes.

Older clients also lose colour tone from their skin, so very few have naturally rosy cheeks; any redness is often caused by broken veins or cosmetic make-up. Dark or ashen colours can therefore be very ageing on older clients who, wishing to look younger, may want to return to the natural hair colour of their youth. Unfortunately this does not always suit them as they get older.

Client lifestyles

The client's lifestyle, occupation and personality is very important.

Lifestyle
The client could be a young working mother, who will not have much time to spend on her hair.

Occupation
Some professions, for example the armed forces and catering professions, have strict rules about the length of hair.

Personality
A quiet, shy person might not be as daring with new styles as an outgoing extrovert. Clients are often worried about other people's reactions to a new hairstyle and may say, 'I'm not sure if my husband/wife will like it'.

Style books
Style books are very useful. They can be bought from hairdressing suppliers or you can make your own. You can then adapt any of the ideas you have from the pictures to suit your individual client.

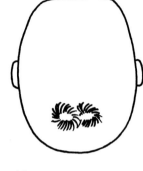

Double crown

TO DO

Make your own style book:
- *buy a plastic folder with clear plastic inserts to hold cut-out pictures of different styles*
- *illustrate the front cover with your salon's name and logo and your name*
- *organise the style book in sections, e.g. short styles, long styles, styles to show hair colours, styles to show different types of perms, styles for special occasions (parties or weddings), styles to suit different face shapes.*

Hair growth patterns

Hair movement means the amount of **curl** or **wave** already in the hair, but hair growth pattern means the direction in which the hair falls.

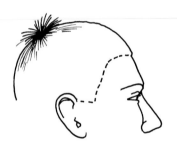

Unsuitable – crown cut too short

This natural fall can best be seen on wet hair. If you comb your client's hair back from the face and gently push the head with the palm of your hand you can see the natural parting falling between the front hairline and the crown.

If you are cutting an all-one-length hairstyle such as a classic 'bob' then you must cut it to the natural parting. Otherwise, when the client tries to do their hair at home, the style could hang unevenly with long ends straying down.

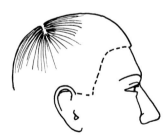

Suitable – longer crown hair

There are several unusual hair growth patterns.

Double crown

If the hair is cut too short on the crown it is impossible for it to lie flat – the hair must be left longer.

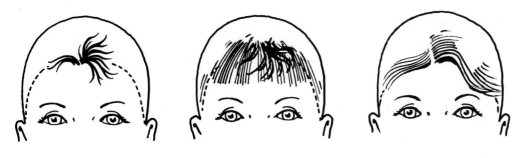

Cowlick

Unsuitable for full fringe

Suitable for uplift fringe

Cowlick

This is found at the front hairline and makes straight fringes on fine hair difficult to cut. It is better to sweep the hair to one side.

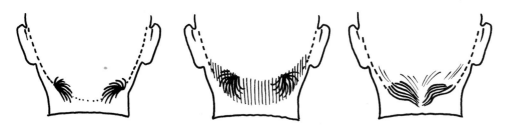

Nape whorl

Unsuitable for short hair

Suitable for 'V'-shaped neck

Nape whorl

This type of hair growth pattern makes straight hairlines difficult to achieve. It is better to cut the hair short into a 'V' shape or grow it longer so that the weight of the hair holds it down.

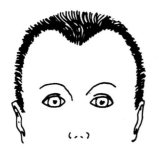

Widow's peak

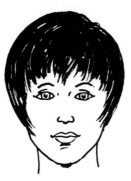

Suitable for heavy fringe

Widow's peak

This is where the hairline grows forward at the front to form a strong centre peak. It is difficult to create a full fringe because the hair tends to separate and lift.

It is better to style the hair back off the face or create a very heavy fringe so that the weight of the hair helps the fringe to lie flat.

TEST YOUR KNOWLEDGE

1 List the different types of hair growth patterns.
2 Describe how a client's lifestyle can affect your choice of hairstyle.
3 Name the four main face shapes and describe a suitable hairstyle for each.
4 Describe how hairstyling can correct uneven head shapes.

Explaining hair treatments to clients

Once you have decided on the type of hairstyle to suggest to your client you should explain it in simple terms. If you went into hospital to have an operation, the doctor would explain what was going to happen to you in clear, non-technical language to make you feel much more confident about what is going to happen to you.

Some clients also feel quite anxious about certain hair treatments such as perming or colouring and need reassurance.

If you explained a conditioning treatment as a 'cationic, deep-acting chemical, which is substansive to the hair, penetrating deep into the cuticle layers and helping to reduce the hair's ability to absorb atmospheric moisture', the client may become somewhat confused!

However, if you said, 'I'd like to apply some of our own deep-acting conditioner to your hair to help the dry, flyaway ends become shinier and more manageable', the client will understand more about the product you are suggesting and why you want to use it.

TO DO

- Look up one method and procedure in this book for perming, colouring and bleaching. Write out a brief explanation of each in your own words.
- Practise explaining the procedures to friends before talking to your clients.

REMEMBER

All hair is porous and can absorb liquids, but over-porous hair or unevenly porous hair is difficult to work with and needs special care.

Hair and skin tests

Whenever you are unsure about how a treatment will turn out you should test the hair first. Hairdressers always use a professional colour chart when selecting a colour so that they do not make mistakes. Testing helps to make both you and the client more confident.

Porosity test

Porous hair can absorb liquids (water or chemicals) through the cuticle and into the cortex.

If the cuticle is closed, flat and undamaged then the hair feels smooth. However, once the hair has been physically or chemically damaged it becomes generally more porous or unevenly porous. This is why special perm lotions are used for tinted and highlighted hair, as normal-strength lotions could quickly over-process or hair colour could become patchy.

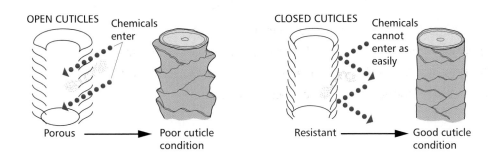

Porous and resistant hair

Method

To carry out a **porosity test**, take a few strands of hair and hold them firmly in one hand near the points or ends and slide your fingers along the hair towards the roots. The rougher the hair feels the more porous it is and the more damaged the cuticle scales are.

> ✂ **TO DO**
> *Practise the porosity test on different types of hair.*

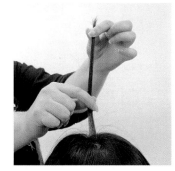

Porosity testing

Elasticity test

Well-conditioned hair is springy and bouncy; this means it has good **elasticity**, and will blow dry or set well. It can stretch up to one-third of its length when dry, half of its length when wet, and then returns to its original length.

However, hair that has lost its elasticity because the internal chemical links and bonds in the cortex have been damaged may stretch up to two-thirds of its length or even break off.

> ✂ **TO DO**
> - *Watch your stylists testing for elasticity when processing highlights.*
> - *Ask your supervisor if you may be allowed to test for elasticity under supervision.*

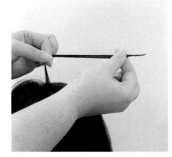

Elasticity testing

Method

To test hair for elasticity, take some dampened hair between your thumb and forefinger and gently pull. If it stretches more than half its length then it is over-elastic and may break off.

Incompatibility test

Some products that clients may have used on their hair may react badly with some of the chemicals that you intend to use – the hair may go green, steam or break off.

The most common products are **hair colour restorers**. They contain metallic salts such as lead acetate and the colour develops over a period of time. The hair often looks slightly greenish and feels harsh to the touch. The problem is that most clients do not admit using them because they do not consider they are colouring their hair (they think they are restoring their natural hair colour).

> **REMEMBER**
>
> Over-elastic hair will be unsuitable for further chemical treatments – cutting and reconditioning should be recommended.

In the salon a client with hair colour restorer on their hair must not have:

- a tint
- a bleach or highlights
- a perm (it is the perm neutraliser that reacts)

because all of these products contain hydrogen peroxide.

If you suspect a client has hair restorer on their hair, carry out an **incompatibility test**. Some temporary hair colours (colours that wash out of the hair), e.g. glitter sprays, also contain metallic salts and need to be removed.

Method

Mix 40 ml of 20 vol (6%) hydrogen peroxide with 2 ml of ammonia (perm lotion will do) in a glass measuring container. Cut a few hair samples (use hair affected by metallic salts) from an unnoticeable area of the client's head and secure them with either cotton or sticky tape. Place the hair samples in the solution and keep them under observation. Results could take anything from one to 30 minutes to show.

If the hair has changed colour, if bubbles have formed in the solution or if the solution has become warm then there are definitely metallic salts on the hair.

Do not proceed with any hairdressing process that involves using hydrogen peroxide.

REMEMBER

Always wear protective rubber gloves when you are using hairdressing chemicals.

TO DO

- Visit several chemists' shops and make your own list of all the products available that contain metallic salts so that you can remember their names.
- Practise an incompatibility test when the opportunity arises.

Colour test: taking a test cutting

In the same way that you would take a hair cutting for an incompatibility test (from an unnoticeable part of the hair), you can easily test hair to see how it will take a hair colour.

Once the hair **test cutting** is secured by cotton or sticky tape at the ends it can be tested with any of the following:

- **temporary colours** – coloured setting lotions or coloured mousses
- semi-permanent colours – colour that lasts 4 to 12 washes
- **permanent colours** – tints that are mixed with hydrogen peroxide
- bleaches – used for highlights or general **lightening**.

Method

Mix a small amount of your intended product in a tint bowl and make sure that the test cutting is completely covered with product. Read the manufacturer's instructions to check the development time, but remember that the tints and bleaches will need longer than this to develop, because there is no warmth from the head to make them work.

After the development time, rinse off the semi-permanent, tint or bleach products (temporary colours are left on) and dry the test cutting. With the client, examine it under natural light (near a window) and decide whether both of you are happy with the result.

Test cuttings are also useful to show whether the hair will take the colour evenly, especially if it is unevenly porous.

Strand test

A **strand test** is taken while the following products are on the hair to check when the product has developed thoroughly:

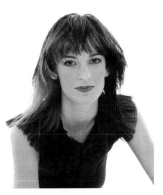

- semi-permanent colours
- permanent colours (tints)
- bleaches
- colour strippers (colour reducers)
- relaxers.

Method
Remove some of the product from a strand of hair with a piece of cotton wool or the back of a comb so that you can see whether it has developed properly, leaving the hair either the correct colour or with the correct degree of straightness.

Pre-perm test curl

This **test curl** is taken if the hairdresser is in any doubt about the likelihood of a perm being successful. If the hair is in poor condition (over-porous or over-elastic) it is better to try out a few curlers first, rather than ruining the client's hair.

Method
Either cut a small piece of hair and tie it with cotton or proceed with a small section of hair on the head. Check with your supervisor when choosing the strength of perm lotion and the appropriate size of rollers to use. Wind the hair around the roller, apply the lotion, develop it for the recommended time, then rinse and neutralise.

If the test is carried out on a hair cutting, once the curl is dry it can either be stored away or shown to the client immediately.

Pre-perm test curls are used to:
- decide the correct strength of perm lotion to use

- decide the correct size of perm curler to use
- determine the amount of time the perm lotion should stay on the hair (**development time**)
- decide whether the hair is in good enough condition to take a perm – if in doubt, take an elasticity test.

TO DO
- *Read Chapter 9 on perming and neutralising.*
- *Watch your stylists perming and make a note of the different steps in the procedure.*

Development test curl

This test is taken when the perm lotion is on the hair during the development process. Once the curl is fully developed the hair is neutralised.

TO DO
- *A development test curl takes a lot of practice and experience, so watch closely when your stylists are carrying them out.*
- *Ask your supervisor if you may be allowed to take a development test curl under supervision.*

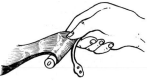

Unwind 1½ turns

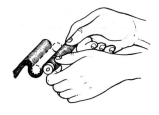

Taking a development test curl

Method

Undo the rubber fastener from one end of the curler. Unwind the curler $1\frac{1}{2}$ turns, without letting the hair unravel completely. Hold the hair firmly, with both thumbs touching the curler.

Push the hair towards the scalp, allowing it to relax into an 'S' shape. Do not pull the hair – remember it is in a very fragile state.

When the size of the 'S' shape corresponds to the size of the curler, the processing can be stopped.

TEST YOUR KNOWLEDGE

State the procedure and the purpose of each of the following tests:

1 pre-perm test curl

2 development test curl

3 test cutting

4 porosity test

5 elasticity test

6 incompatibility test

7 strand test.

Skin tests

Many people suffer from allergic reactions (**allergies**) to food or products (e.g. make-up). Hairdressing is no exception, and clients can become allergic to some hair colours. Permanent colours (which are tints mixed with hydrogen peroxide) and any semi-permanent colours containing **para dyes** always need a **skin test**.

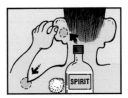

TO DO

Check the instructions on all the types of colours in your salon to see which ones need a skin test.

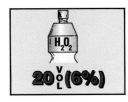

Method

Clean a small, sensitive area of the skin (either behind the ear or in the crook of the elbow) with cotton wool and surgical spirit.

Mix a small amount of the colour to be used with equal parts of hydrogen peroxide, either 20 vol (6%) or 30 vol (9%).

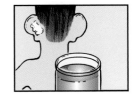

Apply a small smear of the colour (about the size of a 20 pence piece) to the cleansed area.

Allow to dry.

Ask the client to leave the skin test for 24–48 hours, unless there is any irritation, in which case it should be washed off and calamine lotion applied to soothe the skin.

Record which colour and which strength of peroxide you used on a record card, together with the client's name, address and the date.

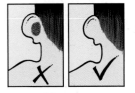

Skin test

Check the skin test when your client returns to the salon. A positive reaction (redness, soreness, itching or swelling) means that your client is allergic to the colour. A negative reaction (the skin appears quite normal when the colour is washed off) means that you can proceed with the colour.

TEST YOUR KNOWLEDGE

State the procedure and the purpose of each of the following tests:

1 Describe how to do a skin test.
2 State the functions of skin tests in predicting reactions.
3 Describe the visible signs of a positive reaction to a skin test.
4 State the significance of a positive reaction.
5 State the significance of a negative reaction.

Consultation checklists

Once you have read this chapter and understand the variations in clients' appearances and hair and scalp conditions you may find the checklist on the following pages helpful for choosing the most suitable products, techniques and equipment to achieve the required look.

REMEMBER

Para dyes are toxic (poisonous) and can cause allergic reactions such as contact **dermatitis** (**eczema**), in which the skin becomes red, swollen, itchy and sore.

Skin tests must be carried out before each application of the hair colour (usually between 24 and 48 hours before). If the client has a positive reaction (redness, blistering, itching, etc.) para dyes must not, under any circumstances, be used.

Other names for a skin test include **patch test**, predisposition test, allergy test, Sabouraud Rousseau test and hypersensitivity test.

Consultation and diagnosis for all salon services

To be used for Unit/Element No _____ Formative/Summative

Date _____ Student's name _____ Client's name _____

☐   ☐   ☐   ☐

tick appropriate box

Client requirements

When was the client's hair last shampooed? _____

Scalp condition Possible disorder/disease _____ Dry/flaky/normal/oily

Hair texture Coarse/medium/fine   **Volume**   Thick/medium/thin

Type African Caribbean/Caucasian/Asian   **Movement**   Straight/wavy/tight curly

Condition Normal/naturally dry/resistant

Previous chemical treatments P/W/relaxed/tint/highlights/lowlights

Hair growth patterns Nape whorl/widow's peak/cowlick/double crown

Testing procedures Elasticity/porosity/incompatibility/strand test/pre-perm test/skin test

Present style Very long/long/medium/short/very short

Layered/graduated/one length/club cut/
razored/clippered/other _____

Client limitations _____

Any additional medical notes _____

Client lifestyle _____

Suggested style _____

Shampoo/surface conditioner recommended _____

Conditioning

Time taken

Name of disorder _____   Product recommended _____

Massage movements _____   Equipment used _____

Cutting

Time taken

With/without fringe   With/without parting   Layered/graduated/one length

Club cut/thinned/razored/clippered/other _____

Styling

Blow dry description _____

Time taken

Tools used _____ Finger dry/natural dry

Set description _____

Roller sizes _____ Pin curls _____

Styling products _____

Finishing products _____

Chemical treatments

Perming Virgin hair/tinted/bleached

Time taken

Pre-condition? _____ If yes, which product? _____

Rod size _____ How many? _____ Winding method _____

Lotion type and strength _____

Processing time _____ With/without heat

Time taken

Neutraliser Type _____ Method _____

Conditioning products _____

Relaxing

Time taken

Product _____

Method _____

Processing time _____

Colouring

Natural hair colour depth _____ % of white _____

Time taken

Temporary/semi-permanent/quasi-permanent/permanent tint bleaching/lightening

Full head/regrowth/partial head

Product name and shade no _____ Peroxide strength _____

Method of application _____

Development time _____

Conditioning products _____

Time taken

Barbering

Beard shape _____ With/without moustache With/without sideburns

Presence of male pattern baldness _____

Additional services recommended to client _____

Additional products recommended to client _____

Client statement

Did the stylist discuss with you your requirements before any services began? _____

Was advice given for your hair and scalp care? _____

Did the stylist recommend products? _____

Will you consider following the recommendations? _____

Stylist signature _____

Client signature _____

Assessor signature _____

Sample questions for clients

Here are some examples of questions to ask your clients:

- 'How often do you shampoo your hair?' If the answer is 'every day' then the client probably has greasy hair and scalp.
- 'How have you been lately?' This gives the client a chance to tell you if they are taking any medication that may affect their hair condition.
- 'Do you have your hair permed or coloured?' The client can then tell you about any chemicals they may have used on their hair.

TO DO

- *Make your own list of tactful questions to ask the client relating to the consultation checklist.*
- *Check them with your supervisor.*

Equal opportunities

The principle of equality of opportunity is that all are treated fairly and equally, regardless of their sex, race, colour, disability, national, ethnic origin and also marital status.

Ensuring a successful consultation

You will need to win over your client so that:

- he or she comes out with a style which is flattering and their hair is in first-class condition
- you do not lose them to the salon down the road!

Here are some helpful guidelines:

- use colour charts and style books to explain your points
- listen to the client, nodding now and again
- reassure the client and be understanding
- offer alternative, positive suggestions such as, 'Your hair cannot be permed at the moment, but after a series of conditioning treatments, I can perm it in six weeks' time'
- do not use technical language
- use eye contact and smile at the client occasionally
- use the client's ideas to your advantage, e.g. 'I like your idea of a short haircut, but with your natural hair growth pattern at the front [the client has a cowlick], I could create a great flicked fringe if it was left a little longer there'.

TEST YOUR KNOWLEDGE

1 Describe what could happen if you carried out a consultation incorrectly.
2 Whom should you refer to if you are unsure about a client's problem or concern?
3 How does the principle of equality of opportunity affect you when carrying out a client consultation?

To obtain the information you need during a consultation, certain types of questions will need to be asked which will help you clarify and confirm the needs and requests of your clients.

- Rhetorical questions, where the answer is already known, e.g. 'Your hair is very dry isn't it?'
- Leading questions, where you suggest the answer needed and you could give the wrong information, e.g. 'I bet you would prefer a beautiful rich chocolate brown rather than a boring set of highlights wouldn't you?'
- Closed questions, where a limited response is needed. Closed questions are all those starting with do, have, did, are. These questions only require a yes or no answer.
- Open questions, where you allow an expanded response, e.g. questions starting with when, how, who, why, what, where. Answers to these questions will give you more information than closed questions.

TO DO

Prepare one example of each of the following:
- *a rhetorical question*
- *a leading question*
- *a closed question*
- *an open question.*
Try them out on a friend and compare the results.

Selling skills

Communicating with people

You can be an excellent stylist but you will never be a successful hairdresser without good communication skills as well. Clients will return to you again and again if you always do their hair well and make them feel special.

Good communication skills when hairdressing include always being polite, cheerful and listening to the client. Listening requires the skill of being able to weigh up, confirm and recommend information. This is determined by intelligence, motivation and knowing the subject well. Many clients never return to salons because they have been given a lovely new hairstyle, but not the one they asked for!

TO DO

Read the section, 'Problems can happen', on page 47. Describe to your supervisor how you would cope with a client who had to be kept waiting for an appointment.

Your communications should be easy to understand, clear and delivered in a pleasant manner and tone of voice. Always clarify any communication to ensure that it has been understood.

Clear communication enhances clients' trust and goodwill. Always clarify any misunderstandings otherwise you can undermine a great deal of careful, thoughtful work. This can be done by:

- advising clients about any delays or disruptions in the service
- looking after clients' belongings careful and reliably
- asking for the help of other competent staff
- recognising cultural differences and requirements.

Communication can be reinforced in the following ways:

- appearance
- posture and body orientation
- gestures and body movements
- head movements
- facial expression
- eye contact
- use of distance and space
- body contact by touching
- non-verbal communication.

Listen with your undivided attention and your clients will feel instantly comfortable. If you are worried about chatting to your clients, try to ask questions that are open-ended, such as, 'How long have you been coming to this salon?' or, 'How do you manage your hair when you go on holiday?' These questions cannot be answered simply by 'yes' or 'no', and so you can start a conversation.

Try to develop a sense of tact. The advice you offer your clients must be passed on in a professional way. Bad atmospheres can often be created by a slip of the tongue, e.g. 'My goodness, you do have bad dandruff'. Confidentiality is also important. If one of your clients suffered from head lice, for instance, the worst thing you could do would be to tell any other clients. Not only would these other clients worry that they might catch head lice, but gossip soon spreads and people might become wary of coming to your salon.

Personal objections must never be aired in the presence of clients as this can ruin the harmony of the salon's working environment. Difficulties must be discussed privately with your line manager.

Verbal communication

All staff members must act in a professional, friendly and helpful manner towards everyone in the salon. Clients should be greeted as per salon procedure with courtesy and respect, e.g. Mr or Mrs, or first name.

Try to increase your general knowledge by reading newspapers or by listening to news programmes on the radio.

Once your confidence is established when dealing with clients, you can start to develop your selling skills.

REMEMBER

Never discuss religion, politics, sex or race with clients, as you can easily cause offence and find yourself in an argument.

Explaining various salon services

All the services that are available in your salon will be displayed on the price list. Clients will often ask about the benefits of different services, and by reading this book you will have already increased your knowledge.

Here are some explanations you might give:
- 'Our reconditioning treatments work particularly well because we give a special massage to help the treatments to penetrate into the hair'
- 'We give two types of permanent waves. One is for a firm curl, which lasts well; the other is an acid perm, which is gentler on the hair and will not dry it out'.

Here is a fuller description of a client discussion.

Discover client needs
Stylist: 'Your hair has some pretty lightness at the very ends. Is that from your holiday last summer?'

Client: 'Yes, the sun lightened it, but it has nearly grown out now.'

Stylist: 'We could always place some natural-looking highlights through your hair to keep it going until next summer.'

Describe features of service
Client: 'Oh yes, how is that done?'

Stylist: 'By using either cap highlights or **foil**. The cap method is quicker and less expensive, but the foil gives more highlights exactly where you want them, and you can vary the colour.'

Client: 'What sort of colour would you suggest?'

Look for buying signals
Stylist: [Uses shade cards] 'These light beige blonde tones exactly match the ends of your hair and would look very natural.'

Client: 'How long do they last?'

Describe benefit to client
Stylist: 'They will grow out gradually, and they give your hair a lot more body, which would help your fine hair keep its style longer.'

Client: 'How much would they cost?'

Close sale
Stylist: 'They are normally £75.00 but we have a special offer for £45.00 if you can make a Monday or Tuesday appointment.'

Client: 'Yes, thank you, I'll make an appointment for next week.'

You can also use style books and product leaflets, rather than just words, to show the client what you mean.

Clients will naturally want to know the cost of the service, so make sure you work it out correctly.

It is also important to explain to the client the length of time involved for different services. For instance, a short cut and blow dry with little hair removed may only take 30–45 minutes, whereas a restyle, cut and blow dry for a client with long hair needing to be cut short may take well over an hour.

Retailing in the salon

All hairdressers have an excellent opportunity for selling products in the salon in that they know what to use and how to use it. Once you have tried your particular salon's mousse, for instance, you will understand its benefits (firm hold, non-sticky, gives lift, etc.) and find it easy to explain these benefits to your clients.

TO DO

Make a short list of each of the products sold in your salon and make a note of:
- *the benefits of each (e.g. normal hold, conditions **dry hair**)*
- *how to use it (e.g. apply to towel-dried hair, apply with your fingertips)*
- *the difference between similar products (e.g. conditioners for permed, coloured or naturally dry hair).*

TO DO

Read the section in Chapter 4 on appointments and make a short list of the benefits, availability, cost and time of the following services
- *cutting*
- *conditioning*
- *perming*
- *styling*
- *colouring*
- *consultations*
- *bleaching.*

You can show the products to clients by the display at the **reception** area, but allowing clients to handle products also helps to sell them. If the client can touch, feel or smell the product – especially when you are using it on their hair – you will always gain their interest.

Understanding your market

You will be selling hairdressing services and hairdressing products to lots of different types of clients, each having various characteristics – long faces, round faces, high hairlines etc. – which make it important for you to recommend the correct product, service and hairstyle for each client.

Here is an example of how to sell a product.

Describe client needs

Stylist: 'Your hair is still a little dry at the ends; would you like me to use our new conditioner today, at no extra charge?'

Client: 'Yes please. What's this one?'

Describe product

Stylist: 'Well, it's one that you actually leave in the hair and don't rinse out. So it does save time.'

Client: 'Won't it leave my hair feeling sticky?'

Stylist: 'Not at all. Try a little on your hands. You can rub it into your skin and see it disappear. It works like that on your hair.'

Client: [Tries the product on her hands] 'Yes, my hands do feel soft and smooth.'

Describe features

Stylist: 'You can use it every time you shampoo your hair and also use it as a hand cream!'

Client: 'How much do I need to use?'

Describe how to use it

Stylist: 'Just squeeze out the size of a small coin, rub the palms of your hands together and smooth the conditioner into the ends of your hair.'

Client: 'Can I buy it at reception?'

Close sale

Stylist: 'Yes, the prices of all the sizes are clearly marked. Remember you get a hair conditioner and a hand cream for the same price!'

Once you have gained some product knowledge, you will find the best way to talk about it is to do it in this order:

1 Describe the product – what it is (e.g. shampoo, **hairspray**).
2 Describe how it works – what it does (e.g. especially benefits permed hair or hair that is washed frequently, or prevents salon colours from fading).
3 Describe how to use it (e.g. hold the hairspray 30 cm away from your hair, or shake the can immediately before use).

TO DO

Re-read the section earlier in this chapter on gowning up, then watch someone do this. Make a note of exactly how to gown up for a perm in your salon.

Here are some examples of client types:
- *young and fashionable*
- *young mothers*
- *uniformed professionals*
- *children*
- *professional business people (e.g. nurses and police officers)*
- *students*
- *senior citizens*
- *European*
- *African Caribbean*
- *Asian*
- *Oriental.*

- *Make a short list of the products and the services that your salon has to offer to suit some of the above client types: e.g. young and fashionable – firm-hold mousse, short clippered styles; senior citizens – regular use of hairspray, firm, curly perms.*
- *Read the sections on 'Tools and equipment' and 'Electrical appliances' on pages 120–126. Make a list of the best types of tools and equipment your clients should buy to use at home and the correct methods of using them, e.g. brushes, combs, hairdryers and other electrical equipment.*
- *Re-read the section on designing a hairstyle to suit your client and make notes on which styles suit different client characteristics, e.g. round face, long neck, etc.*

Developing and responding to non-verbal clues

There are other ways of responding to your client as well as talking to them. This is called body language. It is very expressive and can confirm or suggest the opposite of what is actually being said.

People communicate non-verbally all the time, using both appearance and gestures. It is important that attention is paid to your own body language to ensure that you are pleasant and approachable. For example, someone who stands with their arms crossed can sometimes be seen as being unapproachable. Someone with more open body language will be easier to talk to.

Reading a client's body language is also important throughout the service and clues should be confirmed and/or questioned politely by the stylist.

An important part of communication is listening. This also involves reading body language. Asking questions will confirm that listening is taking place.

Appearances
Hairdressing is all about creating images. Remember, not everyone wants a new hairstyle when they visit the salon. Many clients are quite happy for you to maintain the style they have, with a few possible variations.

Use your common sense when selling services and products. For example, a young working mother with little time to spare would be more willing to buy a combined shampoo and conditioner or a 'wash 'n wear' perm than would a senior citizen with more time on their hands.

Gestures
The obvious gestures that you should look for when selling products and services are as follows.

Head nodding
This means that a client is listening to what you are saying with agreement. A slow, single nod means you should continue what you are saying, and several quick nods mean that the client wants to interrupt and speak themselves.

Eye contact
By looking into someone's eyes you can soon see if they are being friendly or hostile towards you. When you are selling to clients, do look them in the eye while speaking to them to gain their confidence.

Smiling
Simply smiling at clients occasionally will automatically create good humour in the salon. It is very difficult not to smile back at someone who smiles at you!

TO DO

Practise looking in the mirror and keeping eye contact with your client while doing their hair.

TEST YOUR KNOWLEDGE

Describe three good examples of non-verbal communication.

Selling: the three stages

There are three stages to selling.

1 Finding out the client's needs – establish a professional relationship by showing interest and gaining the client's trust as to how you can improve their hair. Identify any previous treatments or problems. You will have learned to do this tactfully during the consultation process. Examples might include fine lank hair; itchy, scaly scalp; dry, split ends. Offer an opinion based on the discussion you have had.

2 Giving the client advice – inform the client of what the product or service will do for them. Explain the benefits, giving examples of them. Ask any relevant questions that will lead you to suggest a particular service or product. Here are some examples:

- fine, lank hair – 'Have you ever thought about having a soft body perm, which just gives volume and bounce?'
- itchy, dry scalp – 'Do you find your itchy scalp becomes worse with certain shampoos?' ('We have one that is especially soothing', etc.)
- dry, split ends – 'How often do you have your hair **trimmed**? We recommend cutting every six weeks to reduce split ends.'

Then offer the product or service.

3 Gaining agreement with the client is achieved either by receiving an immediate response or by giving them time to think about it. For example, 'Would you like a perm on your hair now?' or, 'My hair has been easy to manage with this perm. I'm sure that yours would be too.'

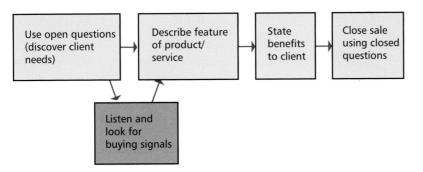

Selling skills flow chart

Finally, do not forget to record any sales or client services on your record card for next time.

TO DO

Using the selling skills chart, practise trying to sell a conditioning treatment, a perm and a colour to a friend in front of your supervisor.
Ask both of them to comment on your performance.

TEST YOUR KNOWLEDGE

1. Using the list of client types, describe both suitable and unsuitable technical services and after-care products for each.
2. Name the particular benefits of giving effective advice to your client.

REMEMBER

If the client has agreed to a further service, write it into the appointment book and confirm it – before they leave!

Salon resources

A hairdressing salon has many resources. Some of them are listed below.

Stock

The stock is mostly hairdressing products, which may be:
- for professional use by the salon staff
- for retail sales to clients.

Fixtures and fittings

Examples of fixtures and fittings are the chairs, the dressing positions (or workstations), the wash-basins, the light fittings and the reception desk.

Utilities

- Power – the electricity supply.
- Water – hot and cold.
- Communication systems – telephones, intercom systems, computers, music systems.

Tools and equipment

This includes hairdryers, accelerators, **scissors**, clippers, razors, combs, brushes, tinting equipment, perming equipment and trolleys.

Time

You are paid for your time *at work*, not just to work on a client's hair and to sit down doing nothing between clients. The salon must be kept clean, tidy and well stocked.

Space

Salon space should never be wasted. For instance, a new delivery of stock must not be left by a stylist's workstation. It should be put into the storeroom immediately so that the workstation is free.

Salon resources are expensive

REMEMBER

All stock is expensive. Always lock storerooms and remove the keys to prevent theft.

Use resources for approved purposes only. Don't use the salon telephone to chat to all your friends, for example.

Try to minimise wastage of stock, utilities, time and space. For example, turn off the lights when not in use and carefully measure out the amount of perm lotion or tint needed for each client.

Make sure you know the security procedures for everything in your salon. In particular, don't leave keys in locks or lying around in the salon and don't leave valuables or products unattended.

Take care not to damage anything in the salon – hairdressing salons are very expensive to equip. If you are not sure how to use something, ask for help.

If you have any ideas about improvements in the salon – perhaps you have noticed that an electrical wire is worn and the wires are exposed – tell your supervisor immediately.

Stock control

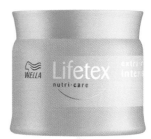

Hairdressing salons cannot run successfully without the correct amount and range of products or stock. However, stock is very expensive and old, unused stock remaining on the shelves wastes money. Existing stock must always be used before new packages are opened to prevent wastage. Using stock in rotation like this is called 'stock turnover'.

Types of stock

Stock for professional use, e.g. perms, relaxers, tints and colours, bleaches, shampoos and conditioners, neutralisers and styling products, is usually kept in a storeroom or a dispensary. Some of the styling products, shampoos and conditioners are kept available for instant use in the salon.

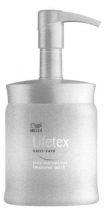

Stock for retail use, e.g. products and sundries (such as brushes, combs, hairdryers, hair ornaments, **wigs** or hairpieces), are sold to clients and the general public.

General stock also includes cleaning products and materials, personal protective equipment such as gowns, towels, protective **capes**, cotton wool, aprons and rubber gloves, and sundries such as tea, coffee, milk and sugar.

Recording stock

Your salon will have a specified method of recording stock levels for salon and retail use.

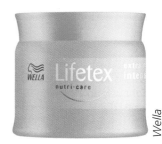

Stock may be recorded on anything from a notepad or a book to a computer.

Wella

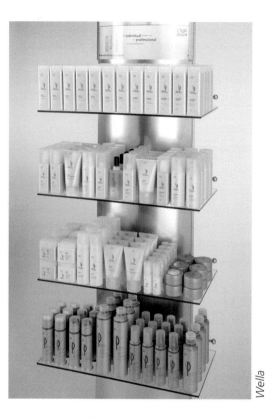

Stock stand

Wella

The following information is normally recorded:

- the date the stock is received
- the name of the supplier
- the quantity and type of stock received
- the value of the order.

Stock records must be checked regularly – this is called stocktaking. Stocktaking is done not only to see what needs to be reordered but also to check which products (or sundries) are selling quickly or slowly.

When you are checking the stock against the records make sure that what you are writing is clear, legible, accurate and complete, as it will be checked by your supervisor.

Stock that has been used is usually checked against the appointment book and the till receipt, giving a double record of where and when it was used. It might be your job to enter the stock delivery in the first place – if you make a mistake there may be problems at a later date if stock was found to be missing.

Stock deliveries

When new stock arrives at your salon:

- unpack it very carefully to avoid damaging the contents. If you are not sure how to open a package properly ask your supervisor
- remove any packaging materials immediately to avoid accidents or untidiness, but check with your supervisor as to how surplus packaging should be disposed of. It may be recycled and not just thrown in the bin!

- check the stock for any damage – this could include crushed boxes, broken lids, or labels peeling off
- look at the sell-by dates – your salon would not want to receive out-of-date stock!
- report any damaged stock immediately to your supervisor, who will deal with the problem and may be able to have the stock replaced
- make sure that the contents match the **delivery note**
- ask your supervisor if you may check the delivery note against the original order
- enter the details of the new stock correctly and accurately into your salon records (often a stock book)
- take the stock to the appropriate place for storage. Remember that all stock must be rotated, which means that old stock must be placed at the front of the storage space and new stock either placed behind it or kept for use at a later date. Products deteriorate after a period of time and will not work properly (e.g. opened bottles of liquid tint become oxidised by the air and will not colour hair successfully).

HEALTH MATTERS

Lifting and carrying heavy stock

Try to use a trolley to transport heavy or bulky items into the dispensary and stockrooms. If the package is too heavy for you to lift, either politely ask another member of staff to help you, or unpack the box carefully until it is light enough to be moved.

When lifting, keep your knees bent and your back straight at all times – you risk straining a ligament or damaging a joint in your spine if you don't lift properly. Keep your feet apart, one foot slightly in front of the other to maintain your balance and face the direction in which the object is to be moved. Never try to lift in a sideways direction. Grip the package firmly, keeping it close to your body, bending your knees and hips, and making sure that your knees are directly above your feet. Allow your strong leg muscles to take the load, not your back.

When lowering the object to the ground be just as careful, keeping your back straight, feet apart and knees and hips bent. Gently does it – lowering heavy objects can be just as dangerous as lifting them.

Sometimes stock needs to be stored on high shelves. Always use a strong, sturdy stepladder, never a chair or anything unsteady.

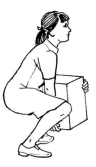 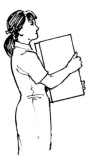

Always lift heavy loads with knees bent and back straight

TO DO

Read the section in Chapter 3 regarding the COSHH Act 1989, 'Storing and using salon chemicals safely'

Displaying stock for retail

Many manufacturers supply special stands for displaying retail stock such as styling products, shampoos and conditioners for home use. As products are sold they should be replaced. You may be asked to restock the stands and to price the products.

- Stock must be displayed safely so that it cannot accidentally fall on anyone (hairdryers are particularly heavy) and out of the reach of children.

- Stock must be displayed in a safe environment at or below room temperature, away from naked flames and sources of heat – particularly direct sunlight. Many products, especially hairspray and nail polish remover, are highly flammable.

- Always check with your supervisor that the product is correctly priced. New stock may be more expensive than older packages of the same product, or the salon may have a promotion or a 'special offer' and be selling stock at a lower price. If you have to stick new price labels on products, make sure the label is clearly visible and does not cover over the name or the contents.

There are two types of retail goods:

- those with a limited life that have a sell-by date (e.g. shampoos, conditioners and styling products). Remember to keep existing stock at the front and place new stock behind it

- products without a limited shelf life (e.g. brushes, combs, hairdryers, hair ornaments, wigs and hairpieces) also need to be sold in rotation in case they go out of fashion.

TEST YOUR KNOWLEDGE

1 Describe your salon's procedure for stocktaking.
2 Why is it important to identify any shortages or surpluses of stock?
3 Why should stock be rotated?
4 Why should stock be displayed properly?
5 List the important points regarding the storage and display of stock relevant to the COSHH Act.
6 Why is it important to use salon resources only for approved purposes?
7 Describe how you could minimise wastage and damage in your salon.
8 Describe the possible consequences of failing to follow your salon's security procedures.

Legislation and retailing

It is useful to have an understanding of the following legislation to help your retailing skills.

Suppliers of Goods and Services Act 1982

This Act is very important within hairdressing, as a hairdresser is a supplier and provider of services and goods. It states that services must be:

- performed with reasonable skill and care
- provided within a reasonable timescale
- provided at a reasonable price.

Goods must:
- be of satisfactory quality
- be fit for the purpose
- match the description given.

When a client asks for a service to be carried out by a stylist a legal contract has been made and as such the client by law has legal rights regarding the service and goods purchased.

Trade Descriptions Act 1968

This Act makes it a criminal offence to either describe goods falsely, or to offer for sale or sell goods that have been falsely described. It not only covers verbal descriptions, but includes advertisements and display cards (by implication, in writing or by illustration), which must also be true and accurate. It applies to services, goods, facilities and accommodation.

The Trading Standards Department of the Local Authority will take enforcement action against serious breaches of the Act.

Consumer Protection Act 1987

Before this Act became law those injured by defective products had to prove a manufacturer negligent before successfully suing for damages. The Act deals with three main areas.

1 Product liability: this is the right of a consumer to sue a manufacturer for injuries or damages caused by defective goods. All products should have a reasonable level of safety.
2 Consumer safety: it is an offence to sell consumer goods that are not reasonably safe in regard to all circumstances (which is why retail hair products such as relaxers are often not as strong as those used in salons). Producers and suppliers must take steps to ensure that they provide the consumer with relevant information and warnings. Hazards must be advertised on a product so that the purchaser can see them. Producers and suppliers must also keep themselves updated about risks.
3 Misleading prices: this covers goods, services or facilities.

The Consumer Protection Act follows European directives to safeguard the consumer from products that may be unsafe.

Disability Discrimination Act 1995 – access to goods and services

This Act states that people with a disability must not be treated less favourably than able-bodied people. Service providers (hairdressers) should consider making reasonable adjustments in their delivery of services to enable disabled persons to make use of them.

Sale and Supply of Goods Act 1994

The terms of this Act state that the seller has to ensure that the goods are:

- of satisfactory quality (as regarded by a reasonable person, having taken into account the description of the goods, the price and any other circumstances that may be relevant)
- reasonably fit – the goods must be fit for their intended purpose (which is why stock rotation is important).

Therefore, goods must be of merchantable quality and fit for their intended purpose (and this includes the conditions under which they may be returned). If they are not, the consumer may be able to claim a refund.

TO DO

Contact the Trading Standards Department of your Local Authority to obtain information leaflets about these five Acts.

TEST YOUR KNOWLEDGE

1 Describe how the Suppliers of Goods and Services Act affects the services and goods that you offer to your clients.

2 How does the Disability Discrimination Act apply to you?

3 What is the main purpose of the Trade Descriptions Act?

4 If a client asked you about a display card describing a new product that you had not been trained to use, why should you ask a member of staff who does know about it to talk to the client?

5 How does the Consumer Protection Act help those who sustain injury from defective products?

6 Name the three main areas covered by the Consumer Protection Act.

7 Describe 'product liability'.

8 Why must hazards be advertised on a product?

9 What is the main purpose of the Trade Descriptions Act?

10 Give four examples of areas covered by the Trade Descriptions Act.

Chapter 2 Performing well at work

After working through this chapter you will be able to improve your personal performance at work by:

- Working effectively as part of a team
- Identifying your own strengths and weaknesses
- Setting and achieving goals
- Understanding appraisals.

This chapter covers the following NVQ Level 2 unit:
Develop and Maintain Your Effectiveness at Work

Introduction

Who are the team members in a salon? They could be:

- other trainees
- junior and senior stylists
- supervisors
- managers
- others working in the salon such as receptionists, beauty therapists, people on work experience, cleaning staff or catering staff.

Salons vary in size – there might be just you and your supervisor in a small salon, you could be part of a medium-to-large salon of 4–20 people or part of a large chain of salons employing hundreds of hairdressers. Wherever you work, you will need to do your own work well, and help and support the rest of the team in an enthusiastic and pleasant manner.

Good staff communication

Many clients return to a salon because it has a good, harmonious atmosphere, and the staff are always happy and cheerful. Tension or bad atmospheres in the salon can result in lost clients and poor working relationships.

To help with a good atmosphere in your salon:

- if someone asks you to help them always respond with a smile
- if you need help yourself, ask for it as politely as you can, even if the pressure is on!
- look and see who needs help in the salon and try to offer support (e.g. passing up perm papers) without being asked first
- don't offer to take on work without checking with your supervisor first (you may think you can attempt a new haircut, but does your supervisor think you can do it?).

Doing your own work well

Here is an example of a technical services checklist. It includes:

- what work you do
- when you did the work
- how you did the work
- where you did the work.

Technical services checklist

Technical Services – Checklist

Your name ....

Type of service – tick   ✓

Cutting	Permanent waving
Drying	Straightening
Dressing hair	Colouring
Setting	Bleaching
	Shaving and face massage

Information required from stylist
MAKE AND TYPE OF LOTION
SIZES OF PERM RODS
WHICH WORKSTATION WILL BE USED

Information required from reception
TIME OF CLIENT ARRIVAL
RECORD CARD

List: Equipment needed
PERM TROLLEY
GREY, BLUE, RED, P/W RODS
END PAPERS
PLASTIC CAP
COTTON WOOL STRIPS
BARRIER CREAM
SECTION CLIPS
PERM GOWNS AND TOWELS
GLOVES

List: Materials/products needed
ACID P/W LOTION STRENGTH
PRE-PERM LOTION
WATER SPRAY
MANUFACTURERS' INSTRUCTIONS

Health and safety notes
CLIENT PROTECTION – GOWNS, TOWELS, COTTON WOOL, BARRIER CREAM
STYLIST PROTECTION – GLOVES
MANUFACTURER'S INSTRUCTIONS, RECORD CARD FOR SPECIAL NOTES
SALON SAFETY – ALL WORK AREAS ARE LEFT CLEAN AND TIDY, AFTER THE EQUIPMENT AND MATERIALS HAVE BEEN PUT AWAY. ANY CHEMICAL SPILLAGES ARE MOPPED UP AND REMOVED.

TO DO

Draw up similar checklists for yourself and complete one for each technical service.

Problems can happen

However well you prepare for the clients, problems can happen! For example:

- clients may be late for appointments (the bus was late, the car park was full)
- clients may arrive without an appointment (regular clients who have suddenly been invited out)
- a new receptionist could have overbooked (two Mrs Greens may turn up for the same appointment)
- a service took longer than the time allowed (the client may have had a complete restyle with their perm)
- the client may have changed their requirement (perhaps the stylist suggested a semi-permanent colour during client consultation for a haircut and it was added to that service)
- a member of staff is suddenly absent due to illness (remember to refer this immediately to your supervisor so that bookings can be rescheduled)
- a client could request an unbooked treatment (e.g. a conditioning treatment) and you could forget to add the cost to the bill
- the wrong record card could be selected and the client could have either a different product (e.g. a colour) or different equipment (e.g. the wrong size of perm rods) used on their hair.

Resolving problems

If there is a problem with the bookings, keep cool, calm and don't appear flustered! Politely ask the client to take a seat while you explain the situation to your supervisor. Your supervisor may suggest an alternative stylist, another appointment or a short wait.

If it is your job to look after the client until their appointment is started, use your initiative. Here are some suggestions of how to use the time:

- explain the delay to the client, giving an indication of how long they may have to wait
- offer the client style books, magazines or newspapers to read
- offer the client tea, coffee or a soft drink
- if the client is not having a chemical treatment, ask the stylist if you may shampoo the client and incorporate a soothing scalp massage (which should take up some of the waiting time)
- if the client refuses to wait and cannot spare the extra time, tell your supervisor immediately, don't wait until the client has left the salon!

> **REMEMBER**
> It is easy to misinterpret instructions while you are in a stressful situation. Always ask for further clarification if you are unsure, rather than make a mistake!

Getting better at your job

Employment rights and obligations for recruitment

It is important to cover the obligations and expectations (rights) for prospective employees at the recruitment and selection stage, so that they have a basic understanding of the fair and legal appointment system and decisions.

Every employee and prospective employee must receive a job description to enable full understanding of the job requirements.

Job description

This describes the main purpose of a job and details the tasks and requirements to do the job. All job descriptions should state:

- job title and location
- main job purpose
- job requirements
- work standard required.

A job description is a useful tool for the employee and employer as it can be used as a measuring tool and a minimum requirement to ensure staff understand exactly what is required of them and also to aid appraisal meetings.

The job description will state your lines of authority, to whom you should report any queries. It will also state any targets that must be achieved and the time scale allowed.

Supporting other team members in their job roles

Many organisations now place a noticeboard at reception with photographs and a brief job description (e.g. manager, artistic director, trainer, stylist, junior, receptionist etc.) underneath. This helps both clients and visitors to the salon identify each member of staff.

Here is an example to help you.

TO DO

Make a line management chart (which should include limits of authority), with everyone's name and position from whom work is allocated. Make a brief summary of each person's job description alongside their names (including your own).

Add a further column which shows your responsibility with regard to being supervised doing that work.

Sample salon organisation chart

NAME	POSITION	JOB DESCRIPTION	LIMIT OF AUTHORITY	MANAGER'S/ SUPERVISOR'S RESPONSIBILITY
Kirsten	Manager	Selection of staff; work allocation; organising staff meetings; organising staff rotas; responsible for salon takings; responsible for staff discipline, providing staff guidance and support, attending to clients	Reports to owner	
Antonella	Senior stylist, long-hair specialist	Staff trainer, attends to clients	Reports to manager (Kirsten)	Planning and reviews of model nights for juniors, planning reviews of staff, long-hair training sessions
Darren	Junior	Trainee (undergoing NVQ Level 2). Assists all staff by shampooing, applying conditioning treatments, neutralising, perm winding, applying colours and blow drying	Reports to senior stylist (Antonella)	Checking Darren's targets and goals through action planning and appraisals

Salon staff are usually given targets within their job role. These can be to achieve per day or per week, or may relate to the amount of money they have to generate per week. Non-achievement of targets are discussed with line management, usually at appraisals. At this time methods of achieving and reasons for non-achievement are discussed and positive encouragement is given.

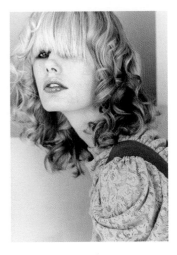

Being able to identify your strengths and weaknesses will enable you to achieve goals. Your line manager will also be able to identify your strengths and weaknesses, and these can be discussed during reviews or feedback. You can identify your own strengths and weaknesses by observing others in the salon performing similar tasks, asking your supervisors and peers, giving questionnaires to clients.

Strengths: what are you good at?
- Is it shampooing, cutting, perming or colouring, for instance?
- Or are client relationships your strength?

Weaknesses: what are your weak points?
- Do you need to improve your technical services?
- Could you improve your speed?
- Could your relationships with the rest of the staff be improved?

TO DO

Make a list of your strengths and weaknesses and go through them with your supervisor.

An action plan should be made to achieve the goal or address the weakness, i.e. what is required to achieve the goal and the time-scale allowed.

Action plans should be reviewed regularly to check progress and they should be amended if required. Action planning is an important tool when improving continuous professional development.

Reviews and feedback

Prepare yourself for a few negative comments from others. It is great to be told that you are better than you thought you were, but sometimes you may not be doing your best. Always accept criticism in a positive manner – remember you are still a trainee, and have much to learn.

Feedback from assessments

The NVQ assessment procedures are ideal for clarifying whether or not your work is up to the required standards. A summative assessment means that you have passed in that area, but you may not have covered all of the range statements – e.g. you have shampooed normal hair above shoulder length, but you still need to shampoo dry, greasy or dandruff-affected hair below shoulder length to complete the assessment.

A formative assessment means that you have not yet passed, and your assessor must explain to you why this has happened – for example, you might not have achieved the desired result, may have used the wrong product or taken too long.

Your supervisor may ask you to agree a target, which may mean, for instance, that in three months' time you will be able to wind a perm perfectly in 45 minutes. It will then be up to you to do enough practice to achieve that target. If you feel that perming is not your strong point, then you could ask for the target date to be set four or five months ahead.

Here is an example of a practical action plan, which helps to focus on your targets.

Practical action plan

Candidate Practical Action Plan

Name: *Tracey Emery*

Start date: *7/9/03*

Date: *23/9/03*

Target outcomes: *Shampooing & Conditioning*

Target date: *18/11/03*

Comments: *I have 1 year's work experience in a salon and need to reinforce my underpinning knowledge.*

Candidate signature   *T. Emery*

Assessor signature   *S. Henderson*

Date:

Target outcomes:

Target date:

Comments:

Candidate signature

Assessor signature

Developments in technology

Hairdressing is a fashion industry that is constantly changing, and to be able to create all the latest styles you must be able to use the most up-to-date tools and equipment and the most recently launched products. You will then be able to offer a full range of services, provide up-to-date advice and promote new services which will generate new business.

Continual professional development/importance of training

Sharing ideas encourages staff development and acquiring technical expertise.

It is important to practise the new trends that develop within the hairdressing industry as success depends on your individual abilities to meet the fast-changing

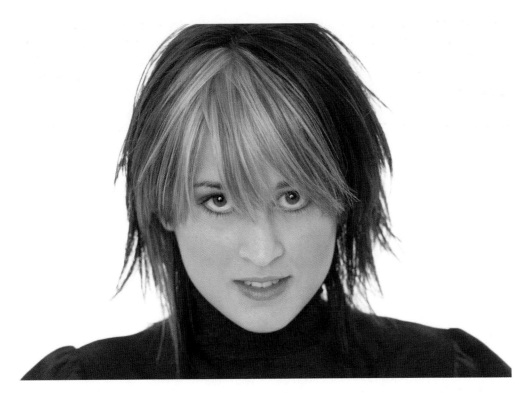

requirements of the industry. Continuous development and training takes place in order for you to:

- increase knowledge
- develop skills
- perform your job more effectively.

There are a number of ways to increase knowledge through training in order to develop and perform tasks more effectively, including the following.

Demonstrations
A look-and-learn method of training.

Job shadowing
Observing a more experienced person doing the task. This is a favourite in salons where trainees can readily observe senior stylists at work.

Training courses/seminars/workshops
Generally consists of a trainer demonstrating new techniques and/or products, and you having the opportunity to put them into practice.

TO DO
Write a description of how to recreate a new technique that you have observed, adding in any sketches or photograhs for future reference.

Both training courses and seminars can be done 'in-house' – at the salon – or outside at a local college/training centre/manufacturer's training school or other suitable venue. To find out when training courses are available ask your supervisor or look in the trade journals such as *The Hairdressers Journal*, *Black Beauty and Hair* or *Estetica/Cutting Edge*.

1 Describe three methods of effectively communicating in the salon that promote harmony within the team.

2 Why is it important that salon staff work in a good, harmonious atmosphere?

3 In what circumstances would you check with your supervisor before starting a task?

4 List all the equipment and materials or products needed for the following technical services:

- cutting
- drying
- dressing hair
- setting
- permanent waving
- straightening
- colouring
- bleaching.

5 Describe the problems that could happen with client bookings and how you would resolve them.

6 In what circumstances would you check with your supervisor for rescheduled bookings?

7 Describe how you could use your time most productively if the salon was not busy.

8 Give two examples of what could happen if you forgot to pass on information to the salon team.

9 What could happen if you offered to take on work without checking with your supervisor first?

10 Describe your strengths and weaknesses for both technical and communication skills.

11 Why is it important to react positively to reviews and feedback from your supervisor?

12 List all the methods by which you could update your hairdressing knowledge, and why this is important.

Chapter 3 # Health, safety and security in the salon

After working through this chapter you will be able to reduce the risks to health and safety in your workplace by:

- Identifying hazards and evaluting the risks in your workplace
- Understanding health and safety legislation and workplace policies
- Behaving in a responsible manner to reduce the risks to health and safety
- Knowing how to deal with emergencies.

This chapter covers the following NVQ Level 2 unit:
Ensure Your Actions Reduce Risks to Health and Safety

Introduction

The following issues are fundamental to working successfully as a hairdresser.

- Hairdressers must always work cleanly. Both your clients' health and your health are at risk. Tools and equipment must be clean and properly sterilised. There are many diseases that you and your client could catch from dirty equipment – such as head lice, impetigo and ringworm. This is known as cross-infection.
- Hairdressers must always work safely. Careless work could lead to hair loss, hair breakage, damage to the client's skin or eyes, or ruined clothes.
- Did you know that legally you (the employee) must take care not only of your own health and safety, but also that of anyone else who may be affected by your work?

This means that you should:

- know where the emergency exits are in case of a fire or bomb alert
- know how to telephone for the emergency services (e.g. the fire brigade, the ambulance service)
- know which chemicals used in the salon are dangerous and how to use them safely
- know how to use electrical equipment safely
- have some knowledge of emergency first aid.

Disease transmission and cross-infection

The prevention of transmitting disease in the salon depends on two main factors:

- good salon hygiene
- the ability of salon staff to recognise which skin and scalp conditions are infectious or contagious and which are not.

Pathogenic bacteria or **micro-organisms** and animal parasites can be transmitted from one person to another. Transmission can take place in two ways: either by contact or indirect contact.

Contact

Touching causes the transmission of the micro-organism or parasite. A disorder passed on in this way is described as being contagious. This contact can be direct or indirect. Touching heads allows the head louse to walk from one head to another; or inanimate objects, which have been in contact with one person and are then touched by another, can spread the disorder. For example, cold sores can be spread by damp towels, face cloths etc., which have been in contact with one person and are then used by another.

Indirect contact

This describes diseases passed on through air or water. When micro-organisms are passed from one person to another in this way it is described as infectious. The micro-organisms that cause the common cold and influenza (flu) are spread by tiny droplets, released by coughing and sneezing, being breathed in by someone else. The micro-organisms that cause **ringworm** (tinea) are often spread in minute skin flakes released by an infected person (or animal).

Cross-infection

Cross-infection can occur if cuts or abrasions are left uncovered, i.e. causing the infection to pass from one wound to another via blood or tissue fluid.

Cuts and abrasions

Open cuts and skin abrasions, particularly on your hands and fingers, and any discovered on your clients, especially on their scalp, neck and face must be considered as serious. Infectious conditions can be transmitted very easily and quickly when blood or tissue fluid from one person comes into contact with that of another person.

Salon hygiene

Preventing the spread of infection

REMEMBER

If you accidentally drop any tools on the floor, clean, dry and sterilise them before using them on the next client. Broken tools must not be used because they can be a source of infection.

- Each hairdresser should have at least two sets of tools, one in use and the other being sterilised or disinfected ready for the next client.

- Clean towels and gowns should be given to each client. Towels should be washed and dried after use (not simply dried).

- Waste hair should be swept up after every haircut and placed in a covered container. Used cotton wool, **end papers** and empty product containers must be placed in waste containers immediately after use.

- All work surfaces must be regularly cleaned with hot water and detergent. Surfaces should be made of materials that are free of cracks and are easy to keep clean.

- Clients with any infectious conditions (e.g. head lice, ringworm or impetigo) should not be treated in the salon but should be tactfully referred to a doctor. If work begins before the problem is noticed, then the service should be completed as quickly as possible. Contaminated hair (e.g. hair with **nits** or head lice in it) should be swept up immediately and preferably burnt – if not, it should be placed in a sealed container. Hairdressing equipment and clothing that has been in contact with the client must be sterilised or disinfected.

- Care should be taken when using tools that may cut or pierce the skin or in areas with open, bleeding or weeping wounds or cuts because of the risk of **AIDS** and hepatitis B (see page 196 on Sharps disposal).

AIDS (Acquired Immune Deficiency Syndrome)

This is caused by a **virus** that attacks the natural defence system of the body so that the person is unable to fight a disease, and this can lead to death. It is transmitted by the infected blood or tissue fluid entering a break in the skin of a healthy person.

Hepatitis B

This is a virus that attacks the liver. Hepatitis is a very serious disease which can kill. It is transmitted by infected blood or tissue fluid coming into contact with the body fluids of an uninfected person, usually through a cut. Therefore combs, brushes etc. should not be used on broken skin affected with boils or skin rashes (such as impetigo) unless they can be **sterilised** immediately afterwards. If you accidentally cut the skin with scissors, clippers or razors, these must be cleaned and sterilised immediately.

Sterilisation and disinfection

All tools such as brushes, combs and hair rollers must be thoroughly cleaned with hot, soapy water to remove loose hairs, dust and **dirt**. Scissors and razors can be cleaned with alcohol. This must be done before sterilisation or disinfection.

Sterilisation

This means the killing of all organisms, whether:

- fungi, e.g. ringworm
- bacteria, e.g. impetigo
- parasites, e.g. head lice.

Autoclaves

These are highly recommended, as they are the most efficient method for sterilising metal tools, combs and plastics (check beforehand that tools can withstand the heat). Autoclaves sterilise by the creation of steam heat (121°C) and pressure, and take about 20 minutes to work.

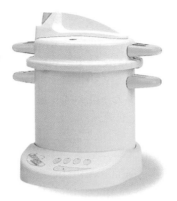

An autoclave

Boiling in water

Towels and gowns should be washed in a hot wash cycle, where the water should reach 95°C.

Ultraviolet radiation cabinet

These **sterilising cabinets** are used in many salons, but all the tools must be perfectly clean before being placed in them. During the process tools must be turned over frequently to expose all surfaces to the **ultraviolet rays**, which come from a mercury vapour lamp at the top of the cabinet. Each side of the tools should be exposed to the ultraviolet rays for 20–30 minutes.

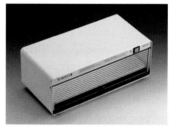

An ultraviolet cabinet

Disinfectants

Disinfectants are effective only if they are used correctly. They quickly become stale or overloaded, and must be used at the correct concentrations for the correct length of time.

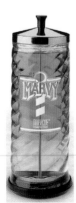

A disinfecting jar

Commonly used disinfectants are:

- hypochlorite – suitable for non-metallic tools and wiping down surfaces. This solution should be made fresh each day
- glutaraldhyde – suitable for metallic tools and wiping down surfaces. This solution can be made up on a weekly basis. Care must be taken to minimise the risk of exposure to this product by ensuring the product is kept closed and that **ventilation** when using is good.

When using disinfectants personal protective equipment such as gloves must be worn.

Personal hygiene and appearance

Salon hygiene is extremely important – but personal hygiene is just as obvious to and necessary for your client.

Think how close you stand to clients when you are doing their hair. Both bad breath and body odour can offend, so keep your breath fresh and remember that soap and water will remove stale sweat, while deodorants (which mask smells) and anti-perspirants (which reduce sweating) can help to prevent body odour.

Strongly flavoured foods and smoking odours can offend clients, so try to steer away from these or use breath fresheners to help combat this.

Keep your hands and fingernails clean and well presented. Be sure to remove large rings and bracelets, which can easily become caught in the client's hair.

Any open wounds must be covered with a waterproof dressing to prevent cross-infection.

TO DO

- *Make a list of the most common infectious conditions that you could contract and pass on in the salon.*
- *Describe where you would go for medical advice for each of these conditions (e.g. to the doctor or to the pharmacist).*
- *Check the list with your supervisor and ask which ones should be reported.*

A hairdresser's style of dress reflects attitudes to fashion and the design of the salon. Accessories such as jewellery, including earrings, brooches, hair ornaments and badges, must blend with the overall look.

TO DO

Make a brief summary of your salon's requirements for personal presentation and conduct.

Generally, clothes worn in the salon should be comfortably loose fitting, clean, neatly pressed and regularly mended. Cotton fabrics are often cooler to wear, but synthetics are generally more hard wearing.

If clients like the way that the hairdresser is dressed and like the hairdresser's own hairstyle, then they will have more confidence in their own finished hairstyle.

When hairdressers look presentable – neat, well groomed and clean – the client will have more confidence and is more likely to return and become a regular client.

Posture

Good posture is important, too, because it looks better as clothes will hang properly. It is also more healthy because the bones, muscles, tendons and ligaments will be held in their correct positions, avoiding undue stretching and strain, which can cause long-term damage to the body.

To stand correctly

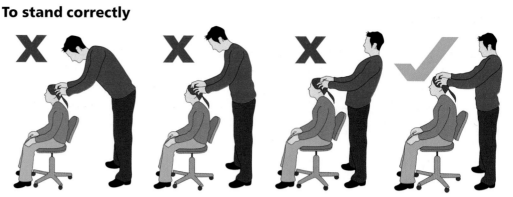

In order to stand correctly keep the feet hip-width apart, with the weight of the body equally on both legs and with the knees slightly bent. Hips and shoulders should be level and the head held up. Common faults are round shoulders, hollow back and weight held mostly on one foot so that shoulders and hips are tilted.

To sit correctly

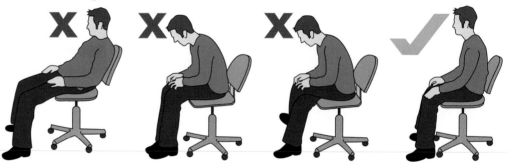

In order to sit correctly the bones should form a right-angle at the hip and knee, with the hips and most of the thighs supported by the chair. Common faults are slouching (only the base of the spine in contact with the chair so that the back and thighs are not supported) and crossing the legs.

Repetitive strain injury (RSI)

RSI is soft-tissue injury caused by repeated motion, i.e. carrying out the same movement over a period of time. It also refers to stress on the body caused by holding awkward or heavy tools over a period of time, and bad ergonomics (using poorly designed tools). Good ergonomics means fitting the task to the person rather than the person fitting the task or job.

RSI can affect anyone whose profession involves continuous, repeated movements of the fingers, hands, wrists and arms within their daily job.

The symptoms include loss of feeling and pain during and after the repeated task. To help reduce the effects of RSI take regular breaks from the task, use the correct posture and exercise frequently.

Feet

Hairdressing demands that a lot of time is spent standing, so it is important to pay particular attention to your feet by wearing comfortable, low-heeled, closed-toed shoes. Cushioned insoles help relieve fatigue. Treat your feet to regular pedicures to help keep them in good order.

Regular exercise

All muscles need to be worked if they are to remain healthy. If unused, muscles will begin to weaken and waste away. Regular exercise, such as running, swimming, aerobics and brisk walking, will keep the muscles working correctly and help to maintain a good body shape. Exercise will also improve respiration, digestion and blood circulation, as well as relaxing nervous tension.

TEST YOUR KNOWLEDGE

1 Why are cleanliness and good hygiene so important in the salon?
2 Name five infectious conditions that may be caught in the salon.
3 What should you do if you accidentally drop any of your tools on the floor?
4 List four points of salon hygiene that will minimise the danger of spreading infection.
5 What is the difference between disinfection and sterilisation?
6 What is the best way to clean and sterilise:

   - towels and gowns
   - combs and brushes
   - scissors?

Safety in the salon

Here is a brief description of the laws that affect you as an employee at work.

Offices, Shops and Railway Premises Act (OSRPA) 1963

This Act says that your salon must be kept safe (against fire, electrical and chemical hazards), and clean and tidy (i.e. hygiene hazards). It means that you have to obey the salon rules.

TO DO

Copies of all Acts and regulations can be purchased from bookshops of The Stationery Office (TSO). Find out where your nearest one is. (You can also purchase such publications online at www.TSO.co.uk.)

All businesses are required to register with their local council.

This Act is being replaced by the Workplace (Health, Safety and Welfare) Regulations 1992, which cover a wider area of health and safety.

Employer's Liability (Compulsory Insurance) Act 1969 and Employer's Liability (Compulsory Insurance) Regulations 1998

These pieces of legislation require employers to take out and maintain insurance on themselves and their employees for accidents to them and to clients. The insurance certificate must also be displayed.

Fire Precautions Act 1971, Fire Precautions (Workplace) (Amendment) Regulations 1997 and Fire Precautions (Workplace) Regulations 1999

These pieces of legislation are enforced by the local fire authority, usually the Fire Brigade. The legislation states that all premises must have fire-fighting equipment in good working order, suitable for the type of fires likely to occur, and readily available. Full training must also be given on the use of the fire extinguishers in the salon premises.

A fire risk assessment of the premises must be performed so that the room contents are arranged and doors left unlocked to enable a quick exit in the case of fire.

Classes of fire

Class A: Fires from solids such as wood, paper, hair etc.
Class B: Fires from liquids such as petrol.
Class C: Fires from gases such as butane and propane.
Class D: Fires from metals.

Types of fire most likely to occur in a salon are Classes A, B and C.

Fire extinguishers

Which portable extinguisher to use	A Freely Burning Materials	B Flammable Liquids	C Flammable Gases	D Flammable Metals	E Electrical Hazards	F Cooking Oil and Fats
WATER	▲					
WATER WITH ADDITIVE	▲					
SPRAY FOAM	▲	▲				
ABC DRY POWDER	▲	▲			▲	
DRY POWDER SPECIAL METAL FIRES				▲		
CO2 GAS		▲			▲	
HOSE REELS	▲					
WET CHEMICAL	▲					▲

Fire extinguisher codes

There are four main types of fire extinguishers that are available for use; these are:

- water – red with a red label, used for Class A fires. Do not use on electrical fires
- foam – red with cream/buff label, used for Class B and small Class A fires. Do not use on electrical fires
- carbon dioxide (CO_2) – red with black label, suitable for all types of fire, especially electrical and Class B fires
- dry powder – red with blue label, suitable for all types of fire, especially electrical, and Class B and C fires. Can damage electronic equipment.

Health and Safety at Work Act (HASAWA) 1974

This Act is enforced by environmental health officers and health and safety inspectors. It protects almost everyone involved in working situations. It requires your employer to:

- provide safe equipment and have safe systems of work
- have systems for the safe handling, storage and transport of products/chemicals
- provide a safe place of work with safe access and egress (exit)
- provide a safe working environment with adequate welfare facilities
- give you all the necessary information, instruction, training and supervision
- provide any personal protective equipment free of charge.

Under this Act the employer has a duty of care towards any other people in the salon, e.g. clients.

Employees have a duty to work so as not to endanger the health, safety or welfare of themselves or others.

It is an offence to interfere with or misuse any items provided in the interests of health and safety, e.g. fire extinguishers, first aid equipment.

All salons must carry out general and COSHH risk assessments (see below) and if your salon employs five people or more (including part-time staff and trainees), the results of the assessments must be written down.

Cosmetic Products (Safety) Regulations 1989

This law covers the rules that recommend different volumes and strengths of hydroxide-based products, i.e. hydrogen peroxide (which is mixed with tints and bleaches and is an ingredient in some perm neutralisers) and relaxers, which are sodium, calcium and potassium hydroxide. Product strengths will vary depending on whether they are made for professional or non-professional (i.e. retail) use.

You can check the product strengths in the manufacturers' instructions and guidance notes. Further guidance can also be obtained by contacting the individual manufacturer or by contacting the Hairdressing Manufacturers' and Wholesalers' Association (HMWA) at: 25 West Street, Haslemere, Surrey, GU27 2AP, telephone 01428 654336.

Environmental Protection Act 1990

This Act states that hairdressing salon chemicals (i.e. 'waste') must be disposed of safely, for example by pouring down the sink (to **dilute** and remove them). Never put them in the dustbin where they could be found by children!

Control of Substances Hazardous to Health Act (COSHH) 1999

This Act is enforced by health and safety inspectors. It is particularly relevant to the storage, use and disposal of hazardous chemicals such as hydrogen peroxide or perm lotions. They must be used in accordance with your salon's rules, the manufacturer's instructions and local by-laws.

The Act applies not only to staff in the salon but also to chemicals applied and sold to non-employees, i.e. clients.

Salons are required to carry out a COSHH risk assessment of the chemicals used and sold in the salon.

The useful leaflet *A Guide to Health and Safety in the Salon*, published by HMWA, is available to all salons.

Electricity at Work Regulations 1989

These regulations state that every electrical appliance in a work site must be tested at least every 12 months by a qualified electrician. A written record must be kept of these tests to be shown to the health and safety authorities upon inspection. You should check the records and testing label dates regularly.

Faulty equipment must be labelled clearly and removed from use until it is repaired.

TO DO

Find the address of your local Health and Safety Executive (HSE) office from the library and contact them to ask for up-to-date publications and information, particularly on fire and evacuation procedures. Or visit www.hse.gov.uk and print off information for health and safety.

Workplace (Health, Safety and Welfare) Regulations 1992

These regulations have replaced most of the Offices, Shops and Railways Premises Act 1963, and require all at work to maintain a safe and healthy working environment.

They apply very strictly to hairdressing salons.

Manual Handling Operations Regulations 1992

These regulations place upon all at work the duty to minimise the risks from lifting and handling objects.

A risk assessment of all manual-handling tasks in the salon should be conducted.

TO DO

- *Re-read the section in Chapter 1 on lifting and carrying heavy stock.*
- *Summarise how best to minimise the risk of injury.*

Personal Protective Equipment (PPE) at Work Regulations 1992

These regulations confirm the requirement for all employers to provide suitable and sufficient protective clothing, and for all employees to use it when required. This means wearing protective gloves and tinting aprons when colouring, bleaching, perming and relaxing. Employees must report damage or loss of personal protective equipment to their employer.

Provision and Use of Work Equipment Regulations 1998

These regulations impose upon the employer the duty to select equipment for use at work which is properly constructed, suitable for the purpose and kept in good repair. Employers must also ensure that all who use the equipment have been adequately trained. The requirement for competence to use salon tools and equipment is embodied within these hairdressing standards.

Reporting of Injuries, Diseases and Dangerous Occurrences Regulations 1995 (RIDDOR)

If you or your clients suffer from a personal injury at work then it must be reported in the salon's accident book. This is to inform your employer and so that serious injuries may be reported to the local enforcement officer.

Some skin diseases such as occupational dermatitis, skin cancer or folliculitis/acne are also reportable and need to be documented for any future reference.

Health and Safety (Display Screen Equipment) Regulations 1992

Employers must provide training on the use of display screen equipment, i.e. computer screens. Breaks when using display screen equipment must also be planned.

Health and Safety (First Aid) Regulations 1981

Employers are required to supply correct first aid equipment and facilities. The amount must be sufficient for the number of staff, who must be able to locate and identify the first aid box.

Management of Health and Safety at Work Regulations (MHSWR) 1999

A risk assessment of the working environment must be performed to measure the safety of staff and clients. The statutory 'Health and safety law – what you should know' poster must be displayed on the premises.

Employers are required to make a suitable and sufficient assessment of the risks to health and safety of their employees and those not employed but who are connected with the business, e.g. clients and visitors.

This requirement is necessary to identify the measures to comply with MHSWR 1999 and HASAWA 1974.

A risk assessment identifies the hazards and the amount of risk involved, including any precautions taken. Action must then be taken to eliminate or reduce these risks and covers everything in the salon, e.g. worn carpet, stairs, fire exits, ventilation etc.

Many of the chemicals and substances used in the salon can be hazardous if they are swallowed, inhaled, absorbed, spilt on the skin or in the eyes or injected. As a hairdresser you should be aware of these hazards, how to prevent them occurring and the recommended treatment if an accident does happen.

This normally includes protective gloves to protect the hands, aprons to protect the stylist's clothing and skin, and gowns to protect the client's clothing and skin. Goggles and face masks could also be provided to protect staff when mixing powder and fume-producing products. Plastic capes also provide waterproof protection to clients.

Every salon must carry out a COSHH risk assessment covering all the products and chemicals used, and explain the results to all the staff. If any personal protective equipment (PPE), e.g. gloves, is found to be necessary as a result of the COSHH assessment this must be provided free of charge by your employer and you must use the PPE.

The procedure for carrying out a risk assessment is the same whether it is a general assessment or a COSHH assessment, as follows.

1 Identify any hazards in the salon.
2 Decide (assess) what the risks are from the hazards.
3 Decide who is at risk.
4 Try and reduce or eliminate the risk.
5 Give all members of staff training to identify hazards and to control risks.
6 Supply any personal protective equipment (PPE) required.

Risk assessments must be reviewed on a regular basis to make sure that they are up to date. Also, a COSHH assessment should be carried out on any new products or chemicals before they are used in the salon.

Example of COSHH Action Plan for salon use

COSHH ACTION PLAN

Date	Problem requiring attention	Priority (High, Med, Low)	Action to be taken	Person responsible	By when Target	Actual	Result
	Staff and clients complaining that perm lotion is causing excessive irritation to the skin	High		Salon manager			Manufacturer can only suggest avoiding skin contact, which is not possible. Product not to be used again. Unused product to be returned for refund.

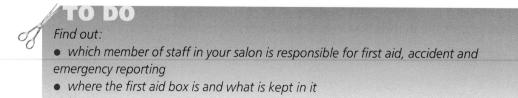

TO DO

Find out:
- *which member of staff in your salon is responsible for first aid, accident and emergency reporting*
- *where the first aid box is and what is kept in it*
- *how your salon's accident book should be completed in the event of an accident or injury.*

Salon hazards

Salon cleanliness is also very important, as there are many ways in which a salon can get dirty or untidy and therefore possible hazards can appear. All staff must be aware of whose job is it to put things right, to clean and tidy up, and to whom to report the hazards.

It is the employees' duty to keep their working area safe. This means that you are ready to act to eliminate possible hazards in the salon. Potential hazards that require further assistance or higher authority should be reported to a senior member of staff.

Carelessness, tiredness or insufficient training can result in accidents such as those listed below.

TO DO

● List all the hazards in your salon and describe how you could remove them within the limits of your own authority.
● Where is the first aid box and what is kept in it?

Accidents in the salon

ACCIDENT	CAUSE
Chemical burns	Spilt hydrogen peroxide Spilt permanent wave lotion or relaxers Use of **incompatible** chemicals (such as metallic dyes and hydrogen peroxide) on hair, creating enough heat to burn the skin, perhaps causing infection and leading to possible legal action by the client Not using barrier cream on the skin
Damage to clothes from products	Not gowning up the client properly and not covering up all of their clothes
Physical burns	Electric tongs, hot brushes, hairdryers, accelerators or infrared bulbs used near the skin
Scalds	Boiling water or steamers burning the skin
Allergies	Permanent dyes (used without a skin test), causing a reaction (contact dermatitis)
Cuts	Scissors, razors (see page 196 for disposing of detachable razor blades), broken glass
Infection	Little or no treatment of injuries Inadequate sterilisation of tools and equipment
Falls	Slippery floors caused by spillage of water, shampoo or grease Obstructions left in the way, such as boxes of stock or large shopping bags
Electric shock	Water and electricity coming into contact Electrical appliances poorly insulated
Poisoning	Drinking from incorrectly labelled bottles Inhaling dangerous vapours from chemicals such as ammonia
Fire	Incorrect handling of inflammable hairdressing chemicals such as ethyl acetate (nail polish remover) and hairspray Careless cigarette smoking

Safety procedures

There are four main areas of salon safety of which you need to be aware:
1 emergency procedures
2 using salon chemicals safety
3 controlling the salon environment
4 using electrical equipment safely.

Emergency procedures

Every salon should have an 'appointed person' who takes charge in the case of an emergency and administers first aid, calls the Fire Brigade, evacuates the building etc. It is important to have procedures for dealing with both fire and other emergencies.

Fire drills should be carried out regularly, at least every six months, to make sure that all members of staff and visitors can be evacuated from the salon quickly and safely. Fire exits should be clearly marked, free from any obstruction, and fire doors must be kept clear from obstruction and be unlocked.

If you discover a fire, inform the appointed person who will raise the alarm, call the Fire Brigade and inform everyone to evacuate the building. Close windows and doors as you leave but don't go looking for personal belongings. If the Fire Brigade are called do not go back into the salon until the officer in charge gives permission.

If it is a small fire, inform the appointed person who will be trained to use a fire extinguisher to put it out.

All electrical equipment should be properly inspected yearly. Plugs should always have the correct size of fuse. Smoking should be limited to certain areas and rubbish should be cleared regularly. Always store any products containing flammable chemicals in a cool place away from direct sunlight as per COSHH requirements.

You must know how to vacate your building quickly and safely in the case of fire, flood, gas leaks, suspicious packages or a bomb alert. You must be aware of where fire-fighting equipment is kept and have been trained on how to use it.

Safety and salon chemicals

Chemical substances become hazardous as a result of:

- inhalation – breathing in fumes
- ingestion – swallowing them directly or by eating food when the chemical is on the fingers
- absorption – through the skin or via the eyes
- contact – with the skin or eye surface (a chemical of this sort is known as an **irritant**).

Basic safety rules for storage of salon chemicals

- Never use food or drink containers to store any chemical product.
- Store products at or below room temperature in a dry atmosphere, never in direct sunlight.
- Keep products, particularly aerosols, away from naked flames or sources of heat.
- Take special care to prevent children gaining access to salon storage areas.
- Keep all products out of reach of children.

Mixing chemicals safely

- Follow the manufacturer's instructions exactly.
- Dilute the product according to the manufacturer's recommendations.
- Never mix products unless this is recommended by the manufacturer.
- Replace all caps and bottle tops immediately to avoid spillage. Make sure unused mixtures and empty containers are disposed of carefully.

Using chemicals safely

- Always wear protective gloves and protective clothing where indicated (see the chart below).
- Remember that prolonged and frequent use of non-hazardous products such as shampoos may cause dryness and sore skin. To avoid this wear protective gloves or use barrier cream and moisturiser as often as possible.
- Wipe and clean all surfaces where spillages occur.

CHEMICAL	HEALTH HAZARD	PRECAUTIONS
All aerosols, including hairspray	Dangerous if inhaled excessively Flammable	Use in a well-ventilated area Keep well away from lighted cigarettes Do not tamper with valves: the contents are under pressure and can explode in a fire
Setting lotions, mousses and gels	Potential irritant Flammable	Avoid eye contact Keep away from lighted cigarettes
Hydrogen peroxide	Irritant to skin and eyes	Always wear protective gloves Avoid contact with eyes and sensitive skin Replace cap immediately after use Do not allow to mix with other chemicals as it can react and become explosive
Bleaches	Dangerous if inhaled excessively Irritant to skin and eyes	Use in a well-ventilated area Wear protective gloves Avoid contact with eyes and sensitive skin
Perm lotions and relaxers	Irritant to skin and eyes	Wear protective gloves Avoid contact with eyes and sensitive skin
Perm neutralisers	Irritant to skin and eyes	Wear protective gloves Avoid contact with eyes and sensitive skin
Hair colours, tints, quasi-permanents and semi-permanents	Irritant to skin and eyes Can cause allergic reactions Always do a skin test before use	Wear protective gloves Avoid contact with eyes and sensitive skin

Controlling the salon environment

This means making sure that the salon does not become too hot or cold or full of dangerous fumes. The Health and Safety at Work Act 1974 states that the working temperature should be 16°C (60.8°F) after the first hour of the salon opening. Precautions should also be taken to avoid high **humidity** in salons due to hair-drying equipment and steam from hot water supplies, which can also make it difficult to work.

TO DO

Find out how to:
- *operate the salon's heating system through the use of thermostats*
- *ventilate the salon by opening the windows or using the extractor fans.*

The COSHH regulations also cover ventilation, especially when mixing chemicals (think about the smell when mixing powder bleach for instance), so make sure you mix products in a well-ventilated area.

Remember that portable gas or paraffin heaters also need proper ventilation to prevent any build up of irritant gases.

Using electrical equipment safely

The Electricity at Work Regulations 1992 state that electrical appliances must be tested regularly for safety by a qualified person, but it is also your responsibility to keep checking that all electrical equipment in the salon is in good condition in order to minimise the risk of accidents involving others and yourself.

- Look at equipment to make sure that the flexes and cables are not worn or faulty. Any flexes with worn insulation or any plugs that are broken or cracked should be switched off from the electrical supply, labelled as faulty and reported to your supervisor.

- Only use electrical equipment for the purpose intended (e.g. do not use electric tongs on wet hair).

- Always make sure that electrical equipment is stable – check that hairdryers, tongs or hot brushes are safely stored on the work surface and not in places where they are likely to fall off.

- Never leave cables (dry flexes) where people could trip or fall over them.

- Check the temperature controls before using any equipment and make sure the filters at the backs of the hairdryers are clear and free of dust or they will overheat quickly.

- Always switch off and disconnect equipment as soon as you have finished with it. Store in allocated areas.

Electric shock

This occurs when a person's body completes an electrical circuit. The size of the shock depends on the size of the electrical current, and can vary from a slight tingling to a cardiac arrest (when the heart stops beating and breathing stops). It can happen:

- when a person touches bare wires on flexes or cables, or uses cracked plugs or switches

- through incorrect wiring, or through a fault in the plug or appliance

- through touching a switch or plug with wet hands – water acts as a good conductor and electricity will flow through the person rather than through the circuit.

Wiring a plug

Make sure you know how to wire a plug correctly.

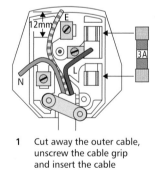

1 Cut away the outer cable, unscrew the cable grip and insert the cable

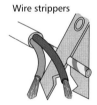

2 Cut away the insulation using wire strippers

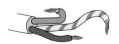

3 Twist the copper strands together

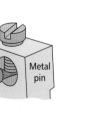

4 Insert each wire into the correct pin

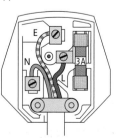

5 Tighten all the screws and the cable grip. Attach the plastic back

Wiring a plug

HEALTH, SAFETY AND SECURITY IN THE SALON

1 Who is responsible for enforcing government legislation regarding accident, emergency and evacuation procedures?

2 Which set of regulations particularly affects:

- obeying the salon rules
- salon insurance
- fire extinguishers for use in the salon
- emergency aid
- the reporting of accidents
- the storage and use of salon chemicals
- disposing of salon waste chemicals safely
- the safety and testing of electrical equipment
- maintaining a safe salon
- lifting and carrying heavy stock
- wearing protective clothing at work
- using display-screen equipment
- ensuring that salon equipment is safe and sound
- risk assessments?

3 Where could you find out more information regarding these laws?

4 What are your responsibilities under COSHH?

5 Why is it important to use safe lifting and handling methods?

6 State your responsibilities under the Health and Safety at Work Act 1974, and related legislation.

7 Why is it important to keep the salon clean and tidy?

8 What could happen if you did not follow the proper evacuation procedures during an emergency?

9 Name four ways in which salon chemicals can be harmful.

10 Why is it important to store chemicals at room temperature?

11 Why is it dangerous to allow children into the stockroom?

12 Why should you always read the manufacturer's instructions before using salon products?

13 Name the chemicals used in the salon for which you always need to wear protective gloves.

14 Which salon products are known to cause allergies in some clients?

15 Which salon products or chemicals are known to be possible irritants to the eyes?

16 Some salon products are known to be more flammable than others. Name them.

17 Why is it important to be able to ventilate the salon properly?

18 Name all the different pieces of electrical equipment used in your salon and list the parts of them that should be tested for safety.

19 What is an electric shock?

20 Give three reasons why electric shock can occur.

21 Why should you always be alert to salon hazards, and to the following in particular:

- spillages
- slippery surfaces
- faulty electrical equipment
- obstructions to access and egress?

22 When should you ask your supervisor to deal with salon hazards?

23 Why is it important to record and report all accidents in the salon?

24 Describe how to dispose of salon waste chemicals and why this is important.

25 Describe the types of records required and how they should be completed.

26 Why is a hairdresser's personal health and hygiene important in the salon?
27 Why is a hairdresser's personal appearance and conduct important to clients?
28 Describe how poor posture and deportment can be harmful to the hairdresser.
29 Name any infectious conditions that may need to be reported in the salon.
30 How should you avoid cross-infection from open cuts and abrasions?

Emergency aid

Emergency aid in the salon usually involves the treatment of minor accidental injuries. However, a qualified first aider would be able to help with more serious injuries such as bone fractures or heart attacks before the patient is seen by a doctor. The aim of first aid is to prevent death or further damage to injured persons. If you have any doubt about an injury, always seek medical advice from a doctor or nurse at a health clinic or the casualty department at a hospital.

Common accidents and conditions in the salon

ACCIDENT/CONDITION	EMERGENCY AID ACTION
Salon chemicals in the eye, e.g. perm lotions, bleaches, tints	Wash the eye with running water (under the tap if possible). Continue applying water to the eye until medical assistance is available
Salon chemicals on the skin, e.g. perm lotions, bleach	Flood the area with water to dilute and remove the chemical
Salon chemicals swallowed, e.g. chemicals placed in soft-drink containers and drunk by mistake	Drink 2–3 glasses of water. Seek medical advice immediately
Salon chemicals inhaled, e.g. strong bleach mixtures	Move the person to fresh air immediately. Seek medical advice if coughing, choking or breathlessness lasts longer than 10–15 minutes
Dry-heat burns, e.g. from hairdryers, tongs, hot brushes, crimping irons	Hold affected area under running cold water or apply ice pack (5–10 minutes). Seek medical advice if necessary
Scalds, e.g. from hot water supplies or steamers	Hold affected area under running cold water or apply ice pack (5–10 minutes). Seek medical advice if necessary
Minor cuts	Apply pressure until bleeding stops. Avoid direct contact with blood because of the risk of infectious diseases such as AIDS and hepatitis B. Wherever possible, ask clients to use a clean piece of cotton wool and apply pressure themselves, then throw the cotton wool into a plastic bag or bin afterwards
Severe cuts	The blood flow from severe cuts should be stopped by applying pressure with either a clean towel or hands (covered with rubber gloves from the first aid box). Phone for an ambulance immediately
Electric shock	If someone is being electrocuted do not touch the person as you will be electrocuted yourself. Turn off the electricity immediately, either by turning off the switches or pulling out the plug. If breathing has stopped then artificial respiration will need to be applied by a qualified first aid person. Phone for an ambulance straight away
Client distress, e.g. fainting	This is caused by lack of oxygen to the brain. If someone feels faint put their head between their knees and loosen any tight clothing. If the person has fainted, raise the legs on a cushion so that they are higher than the head

First aid kits

All salons should provide a first aid box (usually coloured green with a white cross) containing a first aid kit. It should include:

- a first aid guidance card
- individual assorted plasters (preferably waterproof)
- medium, large and extra large sterile dressings
- bandages (including a triangular bandage)
- sterile eye pads
- scissors
- tweezers
- safety pins
- gloves
- saline lotion.

It is also advisable to keep disposable rubber or plastic gloves for dealing with wounds that are bleeding or weeping. Except in an emergency, aid should not be given without wearing these gloves because of the risk of AIDS and hepatitis B.

TO DO

- *Find out where the first aid kit is located in your salon.*
- *Check its contents and report to your supervisor if anything is missing.*

More serious signs of distress, such as heart attacks, stopped breathing, epileptic fits or fractures (from falls), should be dealt with by a qualified first aider. If you wish to qualify, contact your local St John Ambulance which regularly run courses.

TEST YOUR KNOWLEDGE

1. What is emergency aid?
2. When would a qualified first aider be needed?
3. When would you need to seek medical advice or call an ambulance?
4. What items would you expect to find in a first aid box?
5. If perm lotion accidentally ran into your client's eye, what would you do?
6. How would you deal with a child who has accidentally swallowed some hydrogen peroxide?
7. If some bleach spills on to your client's neck, how would you remove it?
8. What is the best treatment for someone who is choking after inhaling a strong chemical?
9. What could cause a dry-heat burn?
10. How should you treat a scald on the hand from boiling water?
11. If you accidentally cut your client's ear, how should the bleeding be stopped?
12. Why must you always wear gloves when treating a person with a severe cut?
13. What is the most important action to take if someone is being electrocuted?
14. Why is it important to raise a person's feet if they have fainted?

Security in the salon

Security of people and possessions

Theft or attack during business hours by salon visitors (such as clients, friends of other staff and business contacts) can be minimised if all staff are trained to establish the identity of all salon callers. Most people will be able to give a valid reason for their visit.

If you approach someone who is acting suspiciously and they cannot give you a satisfactory reason for their visit, alert your supervisor immediately. Do not put yourself at any risk. If the individual runs away, report the incident at once. It is likely that the police will need to be called and therefore you should document the facts. You will need to tell them clearly and accurately:

- the date and time of the incident
- where the incident happened
- what actually took place
- what the intruder looked like.

The police will also require statements from any other witnesses.

The personal possessions of both clients and staff also need protecting from theft. These must be kept safely away from risk situations. Clients' handbags, jewellery and any other valuables should remain with them at all times. Your valuable items or money should be securely stored during working hours, or kept on you, perhaps in your pockets.

Security of salon premises, fixtures and fittings

Salons are often very exposed, having large glass windows and shop fronts. Therefore, do not expose the premises to unnecessary risks, especially by:

- leaving any doors, windows or cupboards unlocked
- leaving money in the till overnight
- leaving valuables in the salon overnight
- not securing all information or data relating to clients and staff.

Security of stock

As far as possible, stock should be available for use as and when required. If you notice any shortages, it may be because there is a thief on the premises.

If most stock is kept in a locked, secure area such as a storeroom, a cupboard or a retail cabinet, the opportunity for theft is minimised. Most salons will have a key holder who has the authority to dispense products, reducing the chance of theft even further.

Stock is a valuable asset belonging to the salon. If your salon has an accurate stock control system, it will be easier to spot discrepancies and shortages.

Unfortunately, theft by salon visitors is not the only way in which stealing occurs. Theft by staff (now often referred to as shrinkage) is something else of which you should be aware. Theft of money, stock or equipment is an act of gross misconduct, and if discovered must be followed by disciplinary action, which may mean instant dismissal.

Security of cash (and cash equivalents)

It is important to maintain a safe and secure environment at the reception area.

All monies must be secured, and products on display must be safeguarded. All personal details of clients, such as record systems, should be held under cover. If a client sees record cards lying around, he or she will have little confidence in the discretion of the salon staff.

To keep reception secure make sure that:

- the reception area is staffed at all times
- all monies are kept secure in the till during the working day
- you never leave the till drawer open when it is not in use or when you have to leave the reception for any reason
- all bank notes are checked to ensure that both the metal strip and the watermark are present. On a forged note, either or both may be missing
- when a client hands you a note, you place it outside the till until you have counted the change accurately
- money is never left in the till overnight
- the till drawers are left open but emptied at the end of the day to prevent a burglar from damaging them by forcing them open
- receipts are given for all payments and bills retained
- all bills, receipts and drawings or additions are noted so that the till will balance.

Regular and random checks

Your supervisor will be taking preventive steps to minimise the risk of theft. Procedures will be set in place to monitor till transactions, stock movements and personal possessions.

Money missing from the till will show up during the daily cashing up. Shortfalls will be noticed when the number of clients attended, services provided and retail stock items sold do not tally with the available money and cash equivalents, the till rolls and totals.

Missing items of stock will be noticed during normal stock control procedures, in routine situations where stock is not available as expected, and during spot checks and searches.

TO DO

- *Make brief notes on your responsibilities for maintaining the security of your salon premises and contents.*
- *Describe how you would report any breaches of security to the relevant person.*

Chapter 4 Reception

After working through this chapter you will be able to run a smooth and efficient reception by:

- Maintaining the reception area
- Attending to clients and enquiries
- Making appointments for salon services
- Handling payments from clients.

This chapter covers the following NVQ Level 2 unit:
Fulfil Salon Reception Duties

Introduction

The reception area not only attracts clients to the salon, but it is also where clients are greeted, appointments are made, the telephone is answered, bills are paid, records are kept, products are sold and clients are gowned up. The busy **receptionist** should look smart, be efficient and capable, and always communicate pleasantly and politely with everyone who enters the salon.

The receptionist will have to:

- greet all clients and visitors with a smile and say, 'Good morning/good afternoon, how may I help you?', then show them where to sit
- make sure the relevant person is informed that the client has arrived
- make all appointments
- answer the telephone
- keep records of salon services (perms, colours, etc.)
- use the cash till to take cash, cheques or credit card payments
- sell products displayed around the salon
- explain the services available to clients
- gown up the clients who are waiting (and organise coffee, magazines, etc.)
- receive deliveries of stock
- keep the reception area tidy by always hanging up the clients' coats in the coat cupboard, removing any gowns left draped over chairs, taking away any used coffee or tea cups, clearing the ashtrays, tidying any piles of magazines, and always making sure that no boxes or bags are left where someone could trip over them
- help clients with their coats and accompany them to the door, checking whether they wish to make a further appointment and making sure that they have collected all their belongings

REMEMBER

Not all salons have a receptionist, so you might have to carry out reception duties as well as being a hair stylist.
Do it well: it is a very important job.
You may also have to deal with electronic enquires at reception. Check with your supervisor to clarify your limits of authority.

- be able to locate the first aid box
- know where the emergency exits are and understand the emergency procedures.

Handling enquiries

Other people, apart from clients and members of staff, who may enter the salon include:

- clients' friends or relatives
- employers' or employees' friends or relatives
- sales representatives.

When these people enter the salon you will need to ask questions, such as:

- the name of the person(s)
- the nature of their business
- the company the person represents
- whom they wish to see
- if they have an appointment booked.

For security reasons always ask for identification, e.g. their company card, since many now include a photo of the person.

The reception desk must never be left unattended, as there could be money in the till, so ask another staff member to go and fetch the person the visitor wants to see.

TO DO

Find out who you should contact in your salon regarding the following:
- *a sales representative*
- *a client with a complaint*
- *a client who wanted to book several appointments on the same day for a wedding.*

Tips for the receptionist

ALWAYS	NEVER
Look like a professional hairdresser: style your hair properly, wear the appropriate clothes and look after your hands and nails	Look untidy: forget to press your clothes, wear laddered tights, wear scuffed, down-trodden shoes, or forget to wear make-up
Act in a professional manner	Smoke, eat, drink or chew gum
Smile, and look at the client, paying attention to what you are doing	Look fed-up or bored or continue chatting with someone else who works in your salon
Sit up properly	Slouch across the reception desk
Greet the client by name (you will know it from the appointment page)	Refer to the client as 'the 2.30', for example
Show the client where to sit	Make clients find their own seats
Apologise to the client if there is any delay	Keep clients waiting without explaining to them that there is a slight problem
Offer the client books, magazines, tea or coffee	Expect clients to help themselves
Deal with any problems in a positive way, e.g. 'I'm sorry, but the last client was a little late, so you may have a short wait'	Look flustered or become aggressive if there are problems. If you cannot deal with a problem, say, 'Would you excuse me for a moment?' and fetch your supervisor

Confidentiality

All details held on clients are and must remain confidential; this means that their information is private and must not be given out. Only authorised staff are allowed to have access to information. Staff details must also remain confidential; this information is only available to authorised senior staff members.

Data Protection Act 1984

This Act places restrictions on the information that can be stored on a computerised data system or on a manual system. It also protects people from having information stored about them without their knowledge.

The Act requires employers using a computerised data system to register as data users. Employers must state:
- that information is being stored on computer
- why it is stored in such a way
- how and from where they have obtained it
- to whom it will be disclosed.

Businesses that store personal details, i.e. client record cards, on computer must register with the Data Protection Registrar and comply with the data protection code of practice.

The Data Protection Registrar must ensure that personal data:
- obtained and processed is done so fairly and lawfully
- is not kept for longer than necessary
- is held only for specified lawful purposes
- is stored in a way that prevents unauthorised access, accidental loss or destruction
- is adequate, relevant and not excessive.

If confidentiality is broken, salon harmony can be affected as trust is broken too. It can lead to loss of business as clients may refuse to revisit the salon. Staff jobs would then be at risk due to someone breaking salon policy and legal action could also be taken against the staff member and salon. Other staff jobs could put be put in jeopardy through loss of business.

Record keeping

Records should be brief, accurate and easy to retrieve.

Recorded information can be stored in two ways:
- writing the information on a record card; or
- entering the information on to a computer system.

The majority of such records in salons are kept as written records. However, many salons use computers to record and store information. A computer will store lots of information and not take up as much room as written paper records.
However, there are some records that should be recorded in a set manner, e.g. recording an accident in the accident book and appointments in the appointment book.

Making appointments

The salon appointment system

Most salons have their own appointment system which is designed to make the best use of the salon's time so that it runs efficiently. Staff workloads are planned on an appointment page, each member of staff has their own work column so that they can plan for the best customer care, especially when several processes are going on at the same time.

Appointment systems also allow for staff to plan their time well and to prepare any products, tools or equipment needed for particular services.

Appointment bookings should be recorded in pencil so they can be removed easily if the booking is cancelled. This allows another booking to be made in its place at the same time.

All handwritten bookings must be clear and neat to enable them to be read with ease. The client's full name or last name and first initial must be legible. Some salons also write the client's telephone number just under their name.

When booking appointments enough time must be allocated for the service, to prevent overbooking and the client having to wait.

When booking an appointment for a client, take the following action:
- existing client – record client name, client record number, telephone number; confirm service required; skin tested if required; confirm appointment with client
- new client – record client name; complete new client record card; register client and client number; confirm service required; skin test given; confirm appointment with client.

Recording appointments

Expected clients, who have already made an appointment, may show you their appointment card or may have made the appointment on the telephone. In either case you need to check the client's name, time and service and the stylist's column on the appointment page. You can then pencil a tick by the client's name, and tell the stylist that the client has arrived.

You must record the same details on the appropriate page for unexpected clients – but you must check first that there is space available.

Always check the appointment details with the client and, if necessary, with the relevent member of staff.

Service abbreviations
These are the abbreviations most commonly used in salons, but there may be others specific to your salon – if in doubt ask.

- C B/D – cut and blow dry
- S/S – shampoo and set
- P/W – permanent wave
- H/L – highlights
- L/L – lowlights
- B/D – blow dry
- C S/S – cut, shampoo and set
- T – tint
- C/T – conditioning treatment.

REMEMBER

Appointments are always made in pencil, so they can be rubbed out if cancelled or changed.

All of these services take different amounts of time. Here is a general guide:

- C B/D – short hair 30–45 minutes
- B/D – short hair 15–30 minutes
  – long hair 30–45 minutes
- S/S – 45 minutes–1 hour
- P/W – 2 hours + drying time
- H/L – 1–1$\frac{1}{2}$ hours + drying time
- T – 1 hour (regrowth only) + drying time.

HEALTH MATTERS

All hairdressers work under the pressure of time, which often results in them working quickly instead of safely. If you can control your own bookings, try to vary the client services, for example, by not doing three cuts in a row, giving your muscles a chance to rest and recover.

The appointment book

Here is an example of an appointment page. You can see here that more time must be allowed for longer processes such as perms and tints.

	GARY	DEBBIE	SHARON
		SATURDAY, JULY 14th	
0830	D. BROWN	G. TEBB H/L (foil)	M. HOWARD
0845	/////// C B/D	/////////////	//////// C B/D
0900	MRS SMITH		J. MOSSMAN
0915	//////// P/W		/////// C B/D
0930	///////////////		A.S. SMITH
0945	MRS JACOB S/S	//////// C B/D	/////// C B/D
1000	MRS SMITH B/D	G. TEBB	
1015	////////////////	//////// B/D	
1030	MRS LOVELL Tint	F. SPENCER	
1045	/////////////////	///// P/W (Restyle)	
1100	G. BRYANT	///////////////	
1115	/////// C B/D		
1130	MRS LOVELL S/S	C. COATES	
1145	A. GREEN	/////// C B/D	
1200	//////// C B/D	F. SPENCER B/D	

REMEMBER

Always allow time for longer processes to be completed, e.g. Gary's column: Mrs Smith P/W at 9.00 a.m. and B/D later (at 10.00 a.m.).

Example appointment page

Appointment cards

Most salons have appointment cards for clients to keep with the salon's name and telephone number and opening times printed on them. When the client is booking in person, once their appointment has been written in the appointment page, complete the appointment card with the date, day, service, time and stylist's name, and then give the card to the client before they leave.

Salon price lists

These are often displayed in the reception area, but some salons also use printed cards. All the prices and services will be listed and it is a good idea for you to learn them.

Sometimes it is difficult to explain a certain price to a client. For instance, someone with long hair needing a cut and perm may be charged more than someone with short hair needing a perm but no cut. If in doubt call your supervisor.

Likewise, do not attempt to give long, elaborate explanations about the benefits of certain processes, such as multicolour foil highlights, until you have been trained to do so. You could give the wrong information. Again, call your supervisor or one of the salon stylists.

Explaining the benefits

Every hairdressing service offered by your salon will benefit the client in certain ways. For example:

- a permanent wave gives more volume, bounce and lift to a hairstyle
- a haircut provides the foundations of a new hairstyle and removes split and damaged ends
- highlights give hair a lighter, brighter appearance, lifting the client's normal hair colour
- a conditioning treatment restores life to damaged, dry ends, giving shine and manageability.

Using the telephone at reception

When you answer the telephone at reception, you must sound professional, courteous and friendly, for instance, 'Hello, this is Headshape. How may I help you?'

sounds much better than 'Yeah?'. You must always identify yourself or your salon and then find out who is calling and what they want to know.

Always replace the receiver properly after receiving or making a call – otherwise your salon will be unable to receive any more calls, and business will be lost.

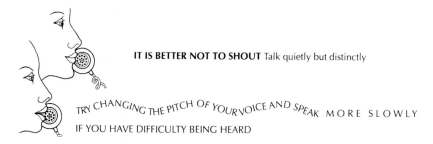

IT IS BETTER NOT TO SHOUT Talk quietly but distinctly

TRY CHANGING THE PITCH OF YOUR VOICE AND SPEAK MORE SLOWLY IF YOU HAVE DIFFICULTY BEING HEARD

Tips for using the telephone

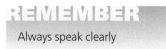

REMEMBER

Always speak clearly

If you are cut off, replace the receiver and wait for the caller to ring again.

Here are some ideas to help you clarify and take down the correct letters and numbers when you are writing out information given over the telephone.

The telephone alphabet

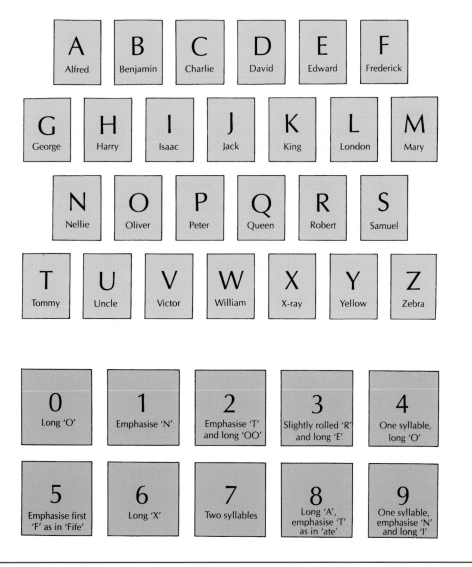

A Alfred	B Benjamin	C Charlie	D David	E Edward	F Frederick
G George	H Harry	I Isaac	J Jack	K King	L London	M Mary
N Nellie	O Oliver	P Peter	Q Queen	R Robert	S Samuel
T Tommy	U Uncle	V Victor	W William	X X-ray	Y Yellow	Z Zebra

Number pronunciation

0 Long 'O'	1 Emphasise 'N'	2 Emphasise 'T' and long 'OO'	3 Slightly rolled 'R' and long 'E'	4 One syllable, long 'O'
5 Emphasise first 'F' as in 'Fife'	6 Long 'X'	7 Two syllables	8 Long 'A', emphasise 'T' as in 'ate'	9 One syllable, emphasise 'N' and long 'I'

Receiving calls

Here are some examples of the reasons people may have for telephoning your salon:

- to make, change or cancel an appointment. Always repeat the message to the person, e.g. 'Thank you, that's Mrs Green, for a perm on Tuesday 2nd April at 1.00 p.m. We look forward to seeing you then'
- to make enquiries about services, e.g. cuts, perms, colours, and their costs
- new clients may call to ask for the salon location and information on where to park their car
- people may call about job availability (you may need to check this with your supervisor)
- hairdressing company representatives (reps) may call to check on an order or to make an appointment to discuss products or equipment
- someone may make a private call to a member of staff. Check the salon policy about this, as some salons will allow emergency calls only and you might have to take a message (see below for more on messages). (There is a sensible reason for this: potential clients cannot make appointments if the line is always busy.) Remember to give the message to the relevant person at an appropriate time. Some messages are confidential, so keep them in a safe place. Disciplinary action may be taken if this confidentiality is broken.

REMEMBER

When taking messages, write down:
- the caller's name
- the caller's telephone number
- a clear message
- the time (and date) of the call.

And pass it on to the right person!

TO DO

Find out your salon's procedure for handling information that is confidential.

Taking messages

It is important that messages are recorded and given to the correct person as soon as possible. This will give a good impression of the salon and will encourage good salon harmony. The main points for message taking include:

- listen with care, with a helpful manner at all times
- write down the message then repeat it back to the sender to ensure it is correct
- ensure the message is written clearly and accurately, making a note of the date and time of the message
- pass the message to the correct person as soon as possible. If the person is not available, let another staff member know that the unavailable person has a message. Remember that every message is confidential
- check that the message has been received and that a reply, if required, has been given.

Making calls

There are three main telephone directories:

- *The Phone Book* (residential and business – listed alphabetically)
- *Yellow Pages* (business – listed by category)
- the *Thomson Directory* (local business – listed by category).

There are three main types of dialling code:

- local codes (you do not need to use one if you are making a call within your local area)

- national codes, e.g. London is 0207 or 0208
- international codes, e.g. 00 is used before dialling the country code for places outside the UK.

TO DO

Use your telephone directory to make a list of the codes for:
- *10 of the largest cities in the UK*
- *10 of the largest countries in the world.*

The Phone Book

You may have to use *The Phone Book* to find the telephone numbers of clients who do not have record cards at your salon. People are listed in *The Phone Book* in strict alphabetical order from A to Z; but, remember, some people choose not to be listed.

You will find the entries set out in the following order: the surname or business name, the initial letter of the first name, then the address. For example:

Abbott A, 21 Roydon Close
Abbott B, 87 Ambrose Ct
Abbott C, 29 Maine Road.

Yellow Pages

- *Yellow Pages* is a directory for business use. For instance, if you need a plumber or an electrician, or if you want to find out where all the other hairdressing salons in your area are, you will find them listed alphabetically by category here.
- There is a *Yellow Pages* for every county. The boundaries of the area covered by each *Yellow Pages* are shown on a map at the front of the book. There is also a list (or index) of categories at the front describing the type of service (e.g. hairdressers) or the goods supplied by the company (e.g. hairdressing suppliers or wholesalers).

TO DO

- *Go through a recent page of your appointment book and make a list of the clients' names.*
- *Check whether these clients have record cards with telephone numbers.*
- *For future use look up the telephone numbers of those not on the records.*

TO DO

Using Yellow Pages:
- *find the number of your nearest hairdressing wholesaler*
- *find the number of your nearest gents' salon, beauty salon and hairdressing school*
- *find the number of your nearest plumber and electrician.*

Operator and telephone engineer services

Dial 100

This operator will help you if you have difficulty in making a call (for instance, if the line is continually engaged and you have tried several times) or if you require special call services, such as transferred (reverse) charge calls or freephone calls.

Directory enquiries

By dialing one of the directory enquiries numbers, which all start with 118 (e.g. 118 118), your call will be answered by an operator who will help you find any UK number or dialling code.

Dial 154

This will put you through to an engineer who deals with faulty lines. Tell them your telephone number and the nature of the fault.

999 calls: emergencies

If an accident happens you should call for assistance immediately.

- Lift the telephone handset and call the operator by dialling 999.
- When the operator answers, tell them the emergency service you want and your telephone number.
- Wait until the emergency authority comes on the line.
- Give the full address of where the emergency help is needed and any important and relevant information.
- Replace the handset.

Never make a false call. It is illegal, and you may be blocking the line for someone who urgently needs the emergency services.

Taking payments in the salon

Calculating the client's bill (including VAT)

Many salons have a sliding scale of charges for the same service, e.g. Salon Directors, Art Directors and Senior Stylists or junior stylists.

When calculating the client's bill, always check if the cut or blow dry/setting service is included in, or excluded from the final charge of a longer service such as colouring, perming or relaxing.

Client's bills are written on a bill pad or a receipt slip, and usually torn off and given to the client to be checked before payment is made.

A typical bill might look like the one below.

		Date _____
Client's name	_____	
Stylist's name	_____	
Service		Price
Cutting		☐
Blow drying		☐
Setting		☐
Permanent waving		☐
Conditioning treatment		☐
Colouring		☐
Bleaching/highlighting		☐
Other services, e.g. manicure		☐
Retail products		_____
	Total	_____
(If applicable VAT is charged at 17.5% of the total cost)	(+ VAT)	_____
	Final total	_____

A typical client bill

Value added tax (VAT)

Many hairdressing businesses have to charge VAT because they are supplying goods and services and exceed a certain income. This tax is then paid to the government at a later date. Some salons include VAT in the price, while others add up the bill and then add on the VAT afterwards.

Example:
Client's bill

Items purchased	Cost	£10.00
	VAT (17.5%)	£ 1.75
	Total cost	£11.75

The percentage rate of VAT (currently 17.5 per cent) is set by the government. It is collected and paid to HM Customs and Excise. It is important that salons keep accurate accounts of monies received and purchases made so that they can calculate the amount of VAT payable to HM Customs and Excise.

Retail items usually have VAT included in the price.

TO DO

Working out VAT is simple with a calculator. If the basic cost of a cut is £10.00, key this amount into a calculator, then + 17.5% and press = and you have the full cost, including VAT, which is £11.75.
- *Using this formula, work out the VAT on the services in your salon.*

Vouchers

Some salons have special offers, gift vouchers or tokens that may be used instead of other forms of payment. Ask your supervisor if these are acceptable in your salon.

Cash payments

The cash till

Cash tills may be electronic or computerised. All tills will have:
- a container for cash or cheques
- a facility for recording the amount taken
- a facility for giving out a receipt.

Giving change

If you always follow the same procedure when giving change you are less likely to make mistakes. If your salon does not have a system you could follow this basic routine.

1 Total the client's bill and tell them the cost.
2 Keep the money the client gives you on the till shelf (do not put the money straight into the till).
3 Count the change into your own hand.
4 Count the change into the client's hand and state how much you are giving.
5 When the client is satisfied that the change is correct, put the money they gave you into the till.
6 Thank the client and give them the till receipt.

REMEMBER
- Always check the amount of cash given to you before you place it in the till.
- Always check the amount of change before you hand it to the client.
- If the bill is very large use a calculator to check that the amount is totalled correctly.
- Always close the till firmly, and lock it if necessary.

Payment by Euro

In 2001, twelve European countries replaced their national currencies with a single European currency called the Euro. Although the United Kingdom has continued to use sterling, some hairdressing salons may decide to accept Euro payments, even though there is no legal obligation to do so. It is important to make sure you know whether or not your salon accepts the Euro so that you can familiarise yourself with the notes and coins.

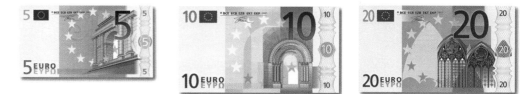

Payment by cheque

If the client is paying by cheque, make sure that it has been completed correctly. If it is not valid your salon will lose that money. Follow this procedure every time you are paid by cheque.

1 Make sure the client has a cheque guarantee card and accept it only if the expiry date (the month and year) has not passed.
2 Check that all of the words and figures are entered correctly on the cheque.
3 If the client has made a mistake, make sure that they have initialled the correction.
4 Check that the account numbers on the cheque card and the cheque (the last group of numbers on the bottom right-hand side of the cheque) are the same, and that the signature on the cheque card matches the one on the cheque.
5 Write the cheque card number on the back of the cheque, then give the client their card and receipt.

TO DO

If you do not have a bank account, ask your parents or close friends if you can examine their cheque guarantee cards. On each, find:
- the account number
- the bank code
- the signature.

REMEMBER

- Always check that you have not taken any foreign money – many banks will not exchange foreign coins.
- Look at bank notes to make sure both the metal strip and the watermark are present. Either or both would be missing from a forged note.
- If there is a shortage of change, tell your supervisor immediately so that the salon does not run out.

A correctly completed cheque

HSBC ◆X◆   400250

Date 11/11/03

Payee *Haringtons*

Date *11th November 2003*

PAY *Haringtons*

Sixty Seventy five pounds £ 75.50

and Fifty pence only————

A. Client

Previous Balance 800

Amount £ 75.50

New Balance 724.50

HSBC Bank International Ltd

Cheque No.   Sort Code   Account No.

123456   400250   23654897

An initialled cheque

Payment cards

If your salon accepts payment cards (Access, Visa and Switch are the most common ones) a sticker will probably be displayed by the door or by the reception desk.

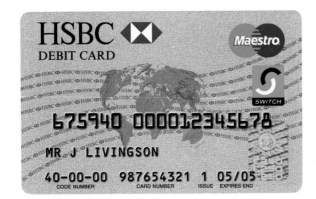

A payment card

Cards can be processed on automated machines (imprinters) that debit the account directly, so that only valid cards can be used. You should pass the card through the machine, then wait until it signals that the card has been cleared and types out the receipt. Ask the cardholder to sign the receipt and then check that the signature matches the one on the card. This is the only check that needs to be done when using this type of equipment.

Follow this procedure if your salon uses an imprinter.
1 Check that the payment card is valid (that the expiry date has not passed).
2 Complete the voucher by writing in:
  ● the date
  ● the hairdressing service (e.g. 'perm', 'cut' or 'blow dry')
  ● the amount to be charged.
  Always use a ball-point pen so that the writing can be seen on all three (carbon) copies.
3 Place the card on the imprinter underneath the voucher, and press down the handle or slide it across so that the imprinter presses the numbers of the card and the name and address of the business on to the voucher.
4 Ask the client to sign the voucher in ball-point pen, then check that their signature matches the one on the card.

5 Give the client the top copy of the voucher as a receipt.

6 Store the other two copies of the voucher safely (perhaps in the cash till); one is kept for the salon, the other will be sent to the card company.

Fraud

Your salon policy will outline the actions to be taken when fraud is suspected. Lines of authority should determine who is to be contacted to help deal with this delicate situation. At all times confidentiality must be maintained and only authorised staff are to be informed.

Over limit – non-cash payments

There may be occasions when a client's bill is over their card limit. In these situations it is important to remain calm and polite and to maintain confidentiality. Your line manager must be informed and they will process the transaction or authorise you to proceed with the transaction.

TO DO

Watch a senior person working at reception when they are:
- *taking a cheque payment*
- *taking a card payment.*

TEST YOUR KNOWLEDGE

(It will help you to re-read the sections in Chapter 1 on client care and communicating effectively with clients.)

1 List three reasons why it is important to communicate well with your client at reception.

2 Name two occasions when you should ask for help from your supervisor while attending to visitors and enquiries.

3 Why is it important to operate your salon's appointment system correctly?

4 List your salon's procedure for taking messages.

5 Messages and record cards are confidential. Give two reasons why this is important.

6 List each of your salon's services and include the cost and time needed for each one.

7 Briefly describe your salon's appointment system, and include:
- the procedures for dealing with expected and unexpected clients
- service abbreviations
- the timing of appointments
- how you should communicate with the member of staff responsible for the scheduled service
- how to take telephone calls and make appointments
- the information needed on an appointment card.

8 Where is your salon's list of retail products and prices located?

9 Describe the forms of payment that your salon accepts. Include the details of an invalid payment and the procedure for dealing with a fraudulent payment.

10 Describe the ways in which you should deal with payment by cash, cheque and credit card.

11 Name two consequences of failing to handle payments correctly.

12 Name two consequences of failing to follow salon security procedures.

Chapter 5 Shampooing and conditioning

After working through this chapter you will be able to:

- Maintain effective and safe methods of working
- Choose and use the correct products for different hair and scalp types
- Shampoo hair and scalp using different massage techniques
- Condition hair and scalp
- Understand the placement and function of certain muscles and bones and tissues of the head and neck
- Prepare hair and scalp for massage services
- Carry out scalp massage using different techniques, tools and products.

This chapter covers the following NVQ Level 2 units:
Shampoo and Condition Hair and Scalp
Provide Scalp Massage Service

Introduction

One of the first procedures learned in the salon is shampooing a client's hair. The client is paying for this service so it must be done properly and better than they could do it themselves.

Reasons for shampooing hair

Clean hair makes you feel great, and a thorough shampoo will remove not only dirt and grease but also hairspray, mousse, gel, setting lotion, flakes of dead skin on the scalp and temporary colours (coloured mousse or colour setting lotions). Tints, bleaches and highlights are also removed from the hair by shampooing.

In the salon, hair is shampooed before styling – and particularly before perming. This is because hairspray, mousse or conditioner on the hair would form a barrier and prevent the perm from taking.

Gowning up

REMEMBER

You may need to observe what the client is wearing when choosing a hairstyle.

After consultation disentangle the hair with a brush or comb at this point. Normally a clean gown, towel and plastic shampoo cape are placed around the client to protect them from any water seeping down on to their clothes.

Positioning the client for shampooing

Various types of wash-basins are used in salons: **back wash**, side wash and front wash.

Back wash and side wash basins

The more popular method involves the client leaning backwards in a chair with the neck resting in the basin's curved recess. The client must be seated comfortably when reclined, with their neck placed centrally in the neck rest of the basin. Most back wash chairs are specially sprung, so when the client leans backwards the back of the chair reclines, allowing them to remain comfortable. The height and position of the chair in relation to the basin is also essential for client comfort. For ideal postitioning for comfort and ease of service, the client should be seated in a near upright position, with the head leaning slightly backwards to prevent water running down the face and to allow the nape area to be cleaned effectively, while the neck is supported in the basin recess.

Back and side wash rinsing is a downward hand movement, with the hand sliding down from the front hairline and covering the ears.

Front wash basins

REMEMBER

The client should be comfortable, dry and relaxed after shampooing; check to make sure.

Tall or short clients, children or people with back problems often require a front wash. The client leans forward facing the basin, a face cloth is held over the eyes to protect the face – particularly from any dangerous chemicals you are using near their eyes (e.g. when neutralising perms or removing bleaches). To avoid wetting the neck and face, forward wash, rinsing using an upward hand movement. It is necessary to control water flow over the neckline by sliding a stretched hand from the base of the neck upwards, so that the water flow is guided up and over the ears.

TO DO

Check with your supervisor on the correct way to gown up a client in your salon for shampooing.

HEALTH MATTERS

Many salons now have free-standing shampoo basins where the shampooist can stand upright rather than leaning across to shampoo the client from one side. The free-standing basins are better because your weight is evenly balanced. If you have to stand on one side, then try to work on one side with one client and on the other side with the next client.

During shampooing try to relax your shoulders and keep your elbows down and in towards your body. Keeping your wrists straight during massage will prevent as much strain as possible.

Most salon shampoos are dispensed from large bottles and the shampoo is forced through a small hole. If this hole becomes encrusted with dried shampoo it becomes even smaller and it is difficult for the shampoo to come out. You may have to strain your wrist and forearm by squeezing hard, so clean the nozzle frequently and keep the container full.

Testing the water temperature

Using the water spray during shampooing takes practice, so test the controls first. Turn on the cold tap first at a moderate rate of flow, then mix in water from the hot tap until the correct temperature is reached. Test the temperature of the water by spraying it on either your wrist or the back of your hand and adjust it as necessary.

TO DO

Practise turning on the water spray to the correct temperature and testing it on your wrist a few times before shampooing your first client.

The hardness of the water

Both water sprays and mixing valves need regular maintenance because **limescale** deposits ('furring up') develop if the water is hard. This can cause blockages and low water pressure, causing hair rinsing to take a long time. Look at the shower spray heads regularly to see if they need cleaning. The head can be cleaned either in place, using a fine pin, or by unscrewing it and using a liquid descaler.

Soft water

If the salon is in a soft-water area, or uses a water softener, then you will not find limescale deposits in water spray heads or 'furring up' in your kettle. Soft water will also lather up easily when you wash your hands with a bar of soap and no scum will be left in the basin.

Hard water

You will know if the water is hard in your area because limescale deposits will be formed around your salon spray heads, in the kettle and in your **steamer** (if you have one).

Hard water contains dissolved calcium and magnesium salts – it is these that produce scum when you wash your hands with soap.

If you have a steamer in your salon it must be filled with distilled water (softened water) so that limescale cannot build up.

TO DO

Wash your hands with a bar of soap in your salon and decide if the water is hard or soft.

Types of shampoo

Soap

A bar of soap or a container of liquid soap is used for washing your hands, not your client's hair. This is because scum is formed from hard-water salts – imagine if the scum that is left in the basin after washing your hands was left in your client's hair!

1 hydrophilic head
(water loving)

hydrophobic tail
(water hating)

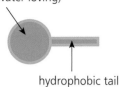

2 dirt and oil

hair shaft

3
detergent
molecule

water molecule
on hair shaft

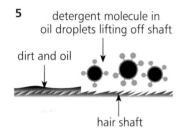

hair shaft

4 detergent molecule in
water on hair shaft

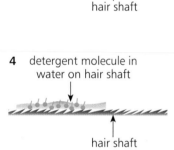

hair shaft

5 detergent molecule in
oil droplets lifting off shaft

dirt and oil

hair shaft

6
water coating
hair shaft

oil in water
emulsion

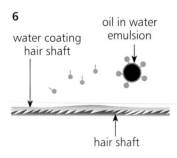

hair shaft

Action of shampoo

Shampoo (for use on wet hair)

Action of shampoos

Shampoos contain **detergents** that help clean the hair by removing the oil and dirt. A detergent molecule is made up of two parts: a head, which is **hydrophilic** (water loving) and a tail, which is **hydrophobic** (water hating).

Detergent also acts as a **wetting agent** by reducing the water **surface tension** and enables the water molecules to wet the hair surface.

Surface tension is a force in liquid surfaces which causes its molecules to pull together and produce a thin film-like layer on top of the liquid surface when in contact with air or other surfaces.

When shampoo is added to wet hair, the hydrophobic tails stick to the grease while the heads stay in the water. The heads repel each other, so the grease is rolled up into round droplets; these droplets are suspended in water as an emulsion, which prevents them from being redeposited on the hair. When the hair is being rinsed, the emulsified droplets follow the water flow – down the drain.

An emulsion = oil and water in solution.

Shampoo ingredients

Many shampoos contain the same ingredients, such as the base detergent or surfactant. This is the washing agent. The base surfactant determines the suitability of the shampoo for the different hair types.

Other additives or ingredients include conditioning agents, e.g. **lanolin** or coconut oil, which have been made water soluble, thickeners such as salt, colours and perfumes, herbal extracts, **solvents**, i.e. lacquer removers, medication, i.e. **zinc pyrithione** (in dandruff shampoo), citric acid to restore the pH value, germicides, i.e. centrimide, and preservatives.

It is the varied amounts of these ingredients that determine which hair type the shampoo is best suited for.

Shampoos designed to restore or correct hair types contain ingredients specially designed and formulated to rectify it, as the ingredient amounts vary in the amount of detergent and emollients. Shampoo containing more detergent and fewer emollients is suitable for fine hair, as it will not leave a heavy residue on the hair, whereas shampoo containing less detergent and more emollients is suitable for **coarse hair**, as this hair type requires softening. It is important to select the correct shampoo for the specific hair type. The wrong shampoo used on the wrong hair type can cause further hair and scalp damage and result in unsatisfactory future salon services, i.e. shampoo suitable for greasy hair used on dry hair will further dry out the hair.

To remove chemical substances from the hair after chemical services, i.e. colours, a shampoo is required that will not affect the chemical process.

If you are unsure about the state of a client's hair and scalp condition always refer to your salon manager who will advise on which shampoo to use.

COSHH – Control of Substances Hazardous to Health Regulations 1999

See Chapter 3 for more details. Alkyl sodium sulphates and ethanolamide or lauric acid are all used in shampoos for their cleaning abilities. Both are known as skin irritants and this is why you must thoroughly rinse all traces of shampoo both from your client's skin and scalp and from your hands. If shampoo accidentally enters the client's eyes, rinse them immediately with sterile water.

Dermatitis

Dermatitis is an **inflammation** or reddening of the skin caused by chemical or physical irritation.

Contact dermatitis

The skin can become dry or damp and itchy. Cracks in the skin can appear and become sore and painful. If left untreated, the condition can worsen and cause deep skin infection. Recommended treatment is prescribed by a doctor. To reduce the risk of dermatitis, which is a common skin condition within hairdressing, always wear protective gloves when providing chemical services. After each service hands should be thoroughly cleaned, dried and moisturised. The application of barrier cream will also help prevent hands becoming irritated and chapped by hairdressing chemicals.

Remember: prevention is better than cure.

If you suspect that you may have dermatitis, you must report this to your manager, as it is a reportable disease (one that needs to be logged in the Accident Record Book and may need to be referred to later if there is an insurance claim or the Health and Safety Executive wishes to investigate).

Always use a barrier cream to protect your skin before and after contact with water and always wear gloves when using chemicals in the salon.

> **REMEMBER**
>
> To avoid shampoo dermatitis:
> - do not wear rings while shampooing
> - rinse and dry your hands
> - use a good hand cream regularly.

Dry shampoos

Sometimes it is impossible to wash a client's hair, for instance if there is no hot water (during a power cut) or if the client has a tender scalp after illness. The hair of such clients can be dry-cleaned (like clothes) by using the following.

- Spirits (alcohol) such as white spirit. Pour the spirit on to cotton wool, rub it onto the hair, then rub clean cotton wool (or a clean towel) over the hair to remove the grease and dirt.
- Dry powders, which are like fine talcum powder. Sprinkle them on to the hair then brush through, allowing them to absorb grease. Dry powders often leave the hair looking dull, so are rarely used in the salon.

The pH scale (acidity and alkalinity)

Hairdressing products, especially perm lotions, relaxers, shampoos and conditioners, often have labels relating to the **pH scale**. Clients often ask, 'Why is an **acid** perm better than an **alkaline** perm?' or, 'Why do some shampoos leave my hair so dry?'. The answers can sound very technical, but it is really quite simple.

The degree of acidity or alkalinity of a hairdressing product can be measured on the pH scale, which runs from pH1 to pH14, where pH7 is **neutral** (neither acid nor alkaline). pH values greater than 7 indicate alkaline substances: the higher the number the more alkaline (and harmful) the product. A pH value less than 7 indicates acid: the lower the number the greater the acidity.

The chart shows that the pH of the hair and scalp is 4.5–5.5, which means they are naturally slightly acid. This is why acid-balanced products are better for the hair and scalp.

TO DO

Research as many hairdressing products as you can find in your salon and local chemist shops to find out which products state the pH and what these pH values are.

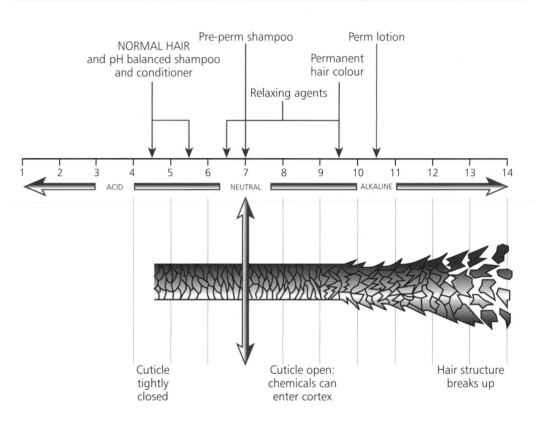

The pH of hair and skin

The diagram of the effect of pH on the hair cuticle shows that acids keep the cuticle scales closed, so the hair looks smooth and shiny. However, alkalis open the cuticle scales, making the hair look rough and dull. Hairdressing processes such as perming, bleaching, tinting and relaxing are all alkaline, because they have to lift the cuticle scale in order to penetrate the cortex and perform their chemical action. Therefore, any conditioning product that has an acid pH (4–6) (an **acid conditioner**) will leave the hair in a shiny, smooth condition.

Strong alkalis destroy the hair shaft (**depilatories**).

Strong acids make the hair harsh and stringy.

To preserve the stable pH value of a product, 'buffers' are added that prevent acidic or alkalinity changes within the product.

The pH of shampoo

Remember that pure water is neutral and will not open or close the cuticle scales. Hair is slightly acid (pH4.5–5.5), so that the cuticle scales are naturally closed.

When you use an alkaline shampoo (pH above 7) the cuticle scales will open, which is helpful before perming as it allows the perm lotion to enter the hair easily.

When you use an acid-balanced shampoo (pH below 7) the cuticle scales will close, which is helpful after bleaching and colouring as it will make the hair shiny again.

TO DO

Take a piece of litmus paper (which indicates pH acidity and alkalinity) and test:
- *all the shampoos in your salon*
- *either a bar of soap or some liquid soap*
- *the water you use to shampoo your clients' hair.*

Choosing the right shampoo

It will be up to you to choose the correct shampoo for your client's hair and scalp type. Always check the manufacturer's instructions – some shampoos have to be diluted, some are left on the hair for a few minutes and some stipulate the need for one or two shampoos.

TO DO

Re-read the sections in Chapter 1 regarding hair and scalp conditions.

Never ask the client to select shampoo they want – you must explain which shampoo (and conditioner) would be most suitable for them.

Normal hair is recognised by:
- being neither dry nor greasy
- not having been permed or colour treated
- holding its style well (good elasticity).

Greasy hair is recognised by:
- the appearance of natural grease on the scalp on a daily basis. Ask when the client last shampood their hair; if it was yesterday or this morning and grease is present it is greasy.

Product build-up (e.g. wax or gel) may make hair look greasy – but this is not greasy hair, and needs a product-removing shampoo.

Dry hair is the most common hair disorder. It is recognised by:
- feeling brittle and dry
- looking dull and rough
- lacking moisture.

Chemically dry hair also feels over-elastic, lacking protein.

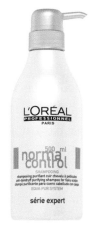

Série Expert Norma Control shampoo – purifying shampoo for greasy hair

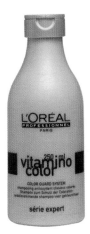

Série Expert Vitamino Color shampoo – anti-oxidant shampoo for coloured hair

REMEMBER

Always check product stock levels and numbers of towels to ensure they are replenished and reordered as required.

HAIR CONDITION	SHAMPOO TYPE
Greasy scalp and hair	Lemon, plain soapless shampoo
Dry scalp with dandruff	Anti-dandruff or medicated shampoo
Normal hair	Moisturising shampoo
Naturally dry hair	Coconut, almond or lanolin shampoo
Chemically dry hair (permed, tinted or bleached)	Protein-conditioning shampoo
Fine, flyaway hair	Volumising shampoo
Hair with excessive hairspray or product build-up	Shampoo with lacquer-removing solvent or product-removing deep-cleansing shampoo
Hair about to be permed in the salon	Plain, soapless shampoo with no additives (these could form a barrier to the perm)
Hair that has just been tinted or bleached in the salon	Acid-balanced shampoo, pH4.5–5.5

Wide-tooth or rake combs

Good for disentangling and combing through products, especially through wet hair as the wide teeth allow hair to pass through, avoiding over-stretching of the hair.

TO DO

- *Match the hair conditions above to a suitable shampoo type found in your salon, noting the ones that need only one shampoo.*
- *Check the results with your supervisor, which includes checking for infections and infestations.*
- *Read the sections in Chapter 3 on the sterilisation and disinfection of tools and equipment.*
- *List and describe four different methods of sterilisation.*

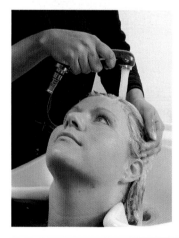

Shampooing the hair

Method for shampooing

Once you have completed your client consultation, positioned your client at the basin, chosen a suitable shampoo (and conditioner if needed) and tested the water temperature you are ready to start.

The effects of water temperature on scalp and hair

The hotter the water during shampooing, the more the scalp is stimulated and the more the cuticle scales will open up, assisting the cleansing process. Therefore, greasy hair should be washed at a lower water temperature so that there is less stimulation of the sebaceous glands. You may need to repeat the shampooing process to remove build-up of products (e.g. hairspray) or if the hair is very greasy or dirty.

Hot water opens up the cuticle scales, and during the shampoo massage procedure, the opened, upturned cuticle scales catch together, producing tangled hair.

Very hot water should never be used when shampooing before perming or before using a semi-permanent colour because of the risk of scalp damage once the chemicals are applied.

Wetting the hair

The hair must always be wetted thoroughly by holding the water spray close to the head and directed away from the face following the different angles of the head. Start at the centre of the forehead, making a barrier with your free hand to protect the client's face from water. Sweep the water over the hair using the spray and hand together. Cup your hand when above and around the ears, patting the water up into the nape hair. Remember to hold the spray until you have turned the water off.

TO DO

Find where the stopcock is in the salon; you never know when you might have a burst water pipe and need to shut the water off.

Applying the shampoo

Never waste shampoo. Look at the amount of hair the client has. A short head of fine hair needs less shampoo than a thick head of long, greasy hair. Use a little shampoo at a time – if you use too much you will have to rinse out a large amount of lather.

Shampoo needs to be applied in several places over the hair, but always pour the shampoo into the palm of your hand first, as this will prevent the shock of cold shampoo on the client's head.

Massage

Starting at the centre of the forehead by the hairline, push your fingers through the hair to the scalp and begin to massage with the pads of your fingers (not your fingernails).

Do not keep your palms flat, but arch your palms and fingers as though you were grasping a large ball. Open and close the whole hand, keeping your fingers well spread and allow the fingers of one hand to pass between those of the other.

When shampoo is spread on to the hair it is called an **effleurage** massage movement. Once the shampoo is evenly applied to the hair you should give a deeper massage – this is known as a **rotary** movement, and helps to thoroughly cleanse the hair. All scalp massage has a beneficial effect in that the blood flow to the skin surface is stimulated, helping to encourage hair growth.

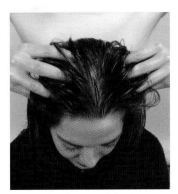

Massaging the scalp

Rinsing

Once you have achieved a good lather, rinse the hair thoroughly until the water runs clear. Check around the front and back hairlines to ensure that no shampoo is left in the hair. Gently squeeze out any surplus water from the ends of the hair.

Thoroughly rinsing shampoo and conditioner from the hair is important to prevent the scalp from drying out due to chemical irritants and to prevent the products from interfering with further salon services.

REMEMBER

If you spill any water or shampoo on the floor, wipe it up immediately to prevent anyone from slipping or falling.

Applying a surface conditioner

If a **surface conditioner** is being applied at the basin, place the required amount (the thicker and more concentrated the product, the less you need) into the palms of your hands and spread evenly through the length of the hair, not on to the scalp. Always check the manufacturer's instructions when using any shampoo or surface conditioner as many have to be left on for 3–5 minutes to be effective.

Combing through conditioner with a wide-toothed comb distributes the product evenly through the length to the ends and makes the hair easier to rinse.

REMEMBER

Only use effleurage on the ends of long, dense hair to prevent tangling.

Disentangling

Use a wide-toothed (rake) comb to disentangle the hair, starting at the ends and working towards the roots so that you do not tear the hair. This returns the cuticle scales to lay in the same direction, away from the scalp. This may be done either at the wash basin or at the dressing position.

Bringing the client to an upright position

REMEMBER

Always check that you have cleaned and tidied the shampoo area before you leave.

There are many variants in the method of using shampoo towels, but what is really important is that the client should remain dry and comfortable.

Bring the client to an upright position when you are ready by asking them to sit up.

Towel drying the hair

Towel-dried hair is hair that is still wet but does not have water actually dripping from it. To **towel dry** the hair hold the towel in both hands, pressing the hair between the two sides of the towel in a smoothing action. The hair is then ready for further processes.

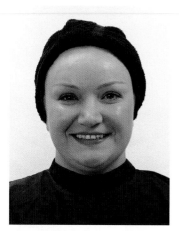

Towel drying the hair

Variations when shampooing

Before perming

Always use a plain, soapless shampoo and do not apply a conditioner before perming as there must be no barriers on the hair.

Two-in-one shampoos, which cleanse and condition the hair at the same time, can cause product build-up on the hair and create a hidden barrier. If the client has been using this product then you must remove it by using a deep-cleansing clarifying shampoo.

After tinting and bleaching

To remove the chemical substances from the hair after chemical services requires a shampoo that will not affect the chemical process afterwards.

Remember, the scalp will be more sensitive after chemical processing, so do not massage too harshly and do not have the water too hot.

REMEMBER

Semi-permanent colours are always lathered then rinsed out of the hair, never shampooed out.

Tints and bleaches have to be rinsed thoroughly from the hair before it is shampooed, twice, to remove all the chemicals. Some tints have a shampoo base in them and will lather up when water is applied.

1 What effects do hard and soft water have on shower spray heads?

2 Describe how the hydrophilic and the hydrophobic parts of a detergent molecule act to clean the hair.

3 Describe how hair condition and subsequent salon services are affected by the pH value of the products used.

4 What effect does an alkaline shampoo have on the hair?

5 Why is it sometimes useful to use an acid-balanced shampoo?

6 Describe the special types of shampoo that would be most suitable for the following:

- greasy hair
- scalps with dandruff
- naturally dry hair
- chemically dry hair
- fine, flyaway hair
- hair with excessive hairspray
- hair about to be permed in the salon
- African Caribbean hair.

7 Give three examples of what could happen if you used the wrong shampoo.

8 Describe the massage movements used during shampooing, and name two occasions when scalp massage should not be used.

9 Would you expect to use more or less shampoo in a soft-water area?

10 Why is it important to always follow the manufacturer's shampoo instructions?

11 Describe three safety considerations to remember during shampooing and conditioning.

12 Why is it important to keep your work area clean and tidy and avoid cross-infections and infestations?

13 What is your responsibility under the COSHH Act during shampooing?

14 What effect does water temperature have on the hair and scalp?

15 On which parts of the hair should you start when disentangling it?

16 Why is it important to remember the direction in which cuticle scales lie when disentangling the hair?

17 What is contact dermatitis?

18 How could you avoid contracting contact dermatitis?

Shampoos for African Caribbean tight curly hair

African Caribbean hair is much drier than Caucasian (European) hair. African Caribbean shampoo contains both mild detergents and higher concentrations of moisturising and detangling agents, creams or oils. A separate oil-based conditioner must always be applied to the hair and scalp after shampooing and left on for three minutes before rinsing. African Caribbean hair that has been chemically treated and is badly damaged needs products containing more conditioning agents that add both moisture (i.e. oils such as coconut, which help to retain moisture) and protein (such as hydrolysed protein or keratin).

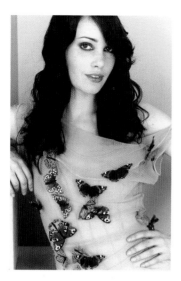

Conditioning

Reasons for conditioning hair

Many clients complain, 'I can't do a thing with my hair at the moment!'. Several things could be causing this.

- Physical and handling damage, e.g. bad brushing and combing, over-drying the hair, excessive use of electrical treatments, excessive tension (elastic bands, tight ponytails), weathering (sunlight, sea and wind).

- Chemical damage, e.g. perming (over-processed perms), relaxing (over-processed hair straighteners), bleaching and highlighting (bleach left on too long), tinting (tint applied on top of tint), use of incompatible chemicals (hair-colour restorers and hydrogen peroxide). Look back at Chapter 1 for more details on how the hair can be damaged.

- Medical history (internal factors), e.g. poor health, poor diet (anorexia often causes hair loss), hormonal changes (pregnancy may cause hair loss and perm failure), courses of medication or drugs (people with cancer may lose their hair during treatment), stress.

You can help to restore the hair and scalp to a healthier state by offering the client a series of conditioning treatments, which, combined with special scalp massages, will also help to relax the client.

TEST YOUR KNOWLEDGE

You will need to remember some facts about the hair and scalp in order to understand how conditioners work.

1 Scalp structure. Label each of the following on diagram A:
   - a sweat gland
   - a sebaceous gland
   - the dermis
   - the epidermis
   - a hair follicle
   - the blood supply
   - a hair
   - the arrector pili muscle.

Diagram A

2 Hair structure. Label the three main parts of the hair on diagram B.

3 Briefly describe the outer layer of the hair, including its colour.

4 Briefly describe the cortex in relation to hair condition.

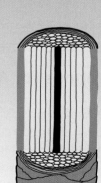

Diagram B

Treating hair and scalp conditions

TO DO

Go back to Chapter 1 and re-read the sections on:
- hair structure
- scalp structure
- non-infectious hair and scalp conditions.

Hair conditions

Fragilitis crinium (split ends)
This is caused by harsh physical or chemical damage. The best treatment is to cut off the split ends.

On dry hair take a small, square section of the damaged hair and twist it. Rub the twisted strand of hair between your thumb and first finger so that the shorter, split ends stick out. These ends are easy to see as they are often white in colour. Hold the twisted hair firmly while you cut off the split ends.

Trimming split ends

Damaged cuticle
The cuticle can be damaged by harsh physical and chemical treatment (remember the pH scale). Once the cuticle scales are raised and the hair feels rough, the hairs will easily matt together and tangle.

Conditioning treatments will help to smooth over and fill in the gaps between the cuticle scales, making the surface appear shiny again. Restructurants will also help to strengthen hair with damaged cuticle scales as they are easily absorbed through the open scales.

Trichorrhexis nodosa
Trichorrhexis nodosa is caused by harsh physical damage (elastic bands) or by chemical damage (e.g. perm rubbers fastened too tightly during perm processing). If the hair can be cut then do so; if not (for example, if the breakage is near the roots) the hair will benefit from reconditioning or restructurants.

Scalp conditions

Pityriasis capitis (dandruff)
There are two basics forms of dandruff:
- loose scale, which leaves the scalp easily
- greasy sticky scale, which builds up on the scalp.

Dandruff is caused by overactive production of the skin cells on the scalp. It is noticeable as small, itchy, dry scales, white or grey in colour. Dandruff shampoos such as selenium sulphide (e.g. Selsun) and zinc pyrithione (e.g. Head & Shoulders®) will lift the skin flakes off the scalp, but should not be used for long periods of time. A few weeks of use should suffice to get rid of the dandruff, then revert to a mild shampoo, using the dandruff shampoos only if the condition recurs.

Dry dandruff may also be treated with oil conditioners or special conditioning creams. Recent reports have suggested that fungicide shampoos (e.g. Nizoral™, which combats any yeasts on the scalp) may also be helpful.

Anti-dandruff treatment

Anti-dandruff treatments should be used infrequently as they slow down renewal of the skin's layers.

Seborrhoea (greasy hair and scalp)

This is caused by overactive sebaceous glands. It is often due to hormonal changes, and teenagers in particular may suffer from it. Seborrhoea can be controlled by shampoos or special spirit lotions for greasy hair. Shampoos designed for greasy hair contain a higher proportion of soapless detergents to remove excess oils.

Generally, advise a client with this condition to avoid stimulating the sebaceous glands, i.e. not to brush the hair too much, not to rub the scalp too much during shampooing and not to use very hot water during shampooing.

Types of conditioner

Oil conditioners

Olive oil, almond oil and coconut oil are pure vegetable oils which can be applied to dry hair then processed with heat. They will make the hair feel soft and supple and look shiny.

Hot oil treatments

Warm oil (used in a process described as a **hot oil treatment**) softens and lubricates very dry or damaged hair.

Acid rinses/pH balancers

These products are balanced with the hair and skin, returning the hair to its natural pH balance of 4.5–5.5.

Weak acids (pH 4–5), such as lemon juice and vinegar (mix one tablespoon to one pint warm water), can be poured through the hair after shampooing and left on. They will make the hair shiny by closing the cuticle scales.

Chemicals, such as neutralisers, bleaches and permanent tints are alkaline (opening the cuticle scales) and they work by adding oxygen to the hair.

Antioxidant conditioners

Antioxidant conditioners stop oxidation, neutralising any alkali chemicals left in the hair and smoothing the cuticle scale.

To return the hair to its natural (acid) state we need to use ascorbic acid. This antioxidant (i.e. it removes oxygen) is often added to acid-balanced conditioners because of its antioxidant properties.

Leave-in conditioners

These contain moisturising and protective ingredients and are sprayed on to wet hair, making it easier to comb. They are ideal for greasy, fine or tight curly African Caribbean hair and are very useful for disentangling children's hair. They also prevent the hair from drying too quickly during cutting, and can be used before blow drying or going out in the sun to prevent damage to the cuticle.

TO DO

List the preparations used in your salon to treat the following conditions:
- fragilitis crinium
- damaged cuticle
- trichorrhexis nodosa
- pityriasis capitis
- seborrhoea.

REMEMBER

Oil conditioners can be difficult to remove from the hair. You must apply shampoo to the oil on the hair, massage to form an emulsion, then apply warm water and rinse.

Conditioning creams (surface conditioners)

Ordinary conditioning creams are emulsions, smoothing the cuticle, easing combing and removing scum, which work in a similar way to the hair's natural grease (sebum). They coat the hair with a thin film, filling in some of the gaps in the broken cuticle scales so normal hair becomes more shiny and manageable. They are applied after shampooing to specific areas of the hair shaft and do not have to be applied to the whole head. They are then rinsed out of the hair. The better ones are acid balanced.

Deep-acting conditioners (penetrating conditioners)

These are sometimes used when reconditioning the hair, especially as a part of a 4–6-week series of once-weekly treatments recommended for chemically treated dry hair in very poor condition and very damaged hair types. They work by rebuilding the internal hair shaft, adding and replacing moisture and nutrients lost. These usually last through a few shampoos and therefore must be applied regularly to keep hair in its repaired condition until it has grown out. They can be applied to specific areas of the hair shaft and do not have to be applied to the whole head.

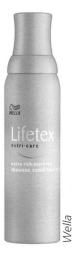

They are usually thicker than ordinary conditioning creams, and stick to the hair better after rinsing (they are **substantive** to the hair and often contain silicones). This is because they are cationic – they have a positive electrical charge, which makes them stick to the hair shaft and remain there.

Products that contain panthenol (derived from vitamin B5) are absorbed into the hair shaft and provide moisture, which helps to retain good elasticity.

Restructurants
Hair that is in a very weakened and over-processed (over-permed or over-bleached) state, such as in trichorrhexis nodosa, will benefit from the application of a restructurant. Restructurants should be applied to shampooed, towel-dried hair and left on (not rinsed off).

Restructurants often contain protein hydrolysates and are sometimes known as protein conditioners (or **penetrating conditioners**). They help to strengthen the hair and can be used before chemical treatments, or for a series of reconditioning treatments.

Conditioning different hair types

Fine or limp hair types
These hair types require light formulas that do not over-soften and are easy to rinse. Apply to lengths and ends, not to the scalp and roots, otherwise hair will be limp and it will be difficult to create volume.

Normal or virgin hair
Such hair may not need a lot of conditioning, but conditioner could be applied to the ends to prevent split ends.

Thick or dense hair
Thick or **dense hair** requires smoothing and softening emollients that can also decrease the volume and make it easy to manage.

Coarse or curly hair
Heavy emollients are ideal to rehydrate dry, rough hair and help define curl.

Chemically processed hair
Reconstructing ingredients are necessary to prevent further damage.

Extra-long hair
Reconstructing products are applied to the lengths and ends; softening ingredients are also applied along the hair lengths to detangle.

When to apply conditioners for chemical processes

Before chemical processing – protective conditioner
Hair that is in poor condition may need either a special type of restructurant or, in the case of perming, a pre-perm conditioner.

Damaged hair is often more porous and will absorb perm lotion very quickly. Some hair is unevenly porous in places, for example on the ends, and may need a pre-perm lotion applied specifically to those areas to even out the porosity.

After chemical processing – corrective conditioner
Acid-balanced conditioning creams are particularly good after perming, bleaching and tinting because they help to replace lost moisture, close down the cuticle scales, work as antioxidants and return the hair to its natural pH balance.

Application of conditioners

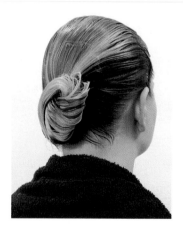

Application of conditioner

- Decide whether you are treating the hair or the scalp condition. If it is the hair, then apply the conditioner to the hair. If it is the scalp, apply the conditioner to the scalp.
- Check whether the product needs to be applied to dry or to wet hair. Oils (e.g. olive oil) are applied to dry hair.
- If the product is to be applied to wet hair after shampooing, always towel dry the hair or the product will be diluted.
- Always disentangle the hair and apply the conditioner according to the manufacturer's directions. **Section** the hair and apply with a brush as you would apply a tint.
- Use a rake comb (a wide-toothed comb) to comb the product through the hair, to distribute it evenly along the length of the hair. NB: products used for scalp treatments (e.g. dandruff, seborrhoea) do not need to be combed through the hair.
- Check the manufacturer's processing times. When processing is complete, rinse the product from the hair. Remember that oil conditioners need to be shampooed out.

TO DO
Look at all the conditioning products in your salon and read the instructions to see how they are applied and how long they should be left on the hair.

Scalp massage

Scalp massage is done once the conditioner has been applied. It is very relaxing and should be done in a calm atmosphere.

The structure of the skin

Re-read the section on the structure of the skin in Chapter 1 to remind yourself of the epidermis and dermis. Beneath the dermis is another layer called the subcutaneous layer. It consists of adipose tissue (fat) and areolar tissue. The adipose tissue helps to protect the body against injury and acts as an insulating layer against heat loss, helping to keep the body warm. The areolar tissue contains elastic fibres, making this layer elastic and flexible. Muscle is situated below the subcutaneous layer.

Sensory and motor nerve endings are found all over the body but are particularly numerous on our fingertips and lips. These nerves will make us aware of feelings of pain, touch, heat and cold by sending messages through sensory nerves to the brain.

Skin structure

The function of the skin

Sensation
The skin contains sensory nerve endings that send messages to the brain. These nerves respond to touch, pressure, pain, cold and heat and allow us to recognise objects from their feel and shape.

Heat regulation
It is important for the body to have a constant internal temperature of 36.8 °C. The skin helps to maintain this temperature by the following means.

- Vasoconstriction – occurs when the body becomes cold. The blood vessels constrict, reducing the flow of blood through the capillaries. Heat loss from the surface of the skin is therefore reduced.
- Vasodilation – this occurs when the body becomes too hot. The capillaries expand and the blood flow increases; this allows heat to be lost from the body by radiation.
- Goose bumps – the contraction of the erector pili muscle when we are cold causes our hairs to stand on end, keeping a layer of warm air close to the body. This was probably of more use to our ancestors, who were generally hairier.
- Shivering – helps to warm the body when we are cold, as the contraction of the muscles produces heat within the body.
- Sweating – in hot conditions the rate of sweat production increases. The **eccrine glands** excrete sweat on to the skin surface and so heat is lost as the water evaporates from the skin.

Absorption
The skin is largely waterproof and absorbs very little, although certain substances are able to pass through the basal layer. Essential oils can pass through the hair follicles and into the bloodstream. Certain medications such as hormone replacement therapy can be given through patches placed on the skin. Ultraviolet rays from the sun are also able to penetrate through the basal layer.

Protection

The skin protects the body by keeping harmful bacteria out and provides a covering for all the organs inside. It also protects underlying structures from the harmful effects of ultraviolet (UV) light. The other functions of the skin also help to protect the body.

Excretion

Eccrine glands excrete sweat on to the skin's surface. Sweat consists of 99.4 per cent water, 0.4 per cent toxins and 0.2 per cent salts.

Secretion

Sebum is a fatty substance secreted from the sebaceous gland on to the skin's surface. It keeps the skin supple and helps to waterproof it.

Vitamin D

The UV rays from the sun penetrate through the skin's layers and activate a chemical found in the skin called ergosterol, which changes into vitamin D. Vitamin D is essential for healthy bones and deficiency can cause rickets, a condition in which the bones are malformed.

Effects of massage on the blood circulatory system

Massage causes the blood vessels to be compressed, forcing blood forwards. As pressure is released the blood vessels return to their normal size and blood rushes in to fill the space created. Reddening of the skin, called erythema, results. Fresh, oxygenated blood and nutrients are brought to the area and so will nourish the tissues and help with tissue repair. Waste products (metabolic waste) are removed and carried away by the veins. A build-up of waste products can cause pain and stiffness and so massage can help to relieve these symptoms.

Massage movements such as effleurage (stroking) will help to return the blood in the veins back to the heart (venous return). This is why strokes are performed in the direction of the venous flow.

The lymphatic system

Have you noticed that certain glands swell up when you are ill, such as the glands in the neck, which inflame during a throat infection? The glands you can feel are lymph nodes. Lymph nodes, lymph, lymph vessels and lymphatic ducts all make up the lymphatic system, which is closely related to the blood circulation. Lymph is similar to blood plasma but contains more white blood cells.

The functions of the lymphatic system

- Helps to fight infection – the production of lymphocytes and antibodies by the lymphatic system is an important part of the immune system. Lymphocytes (white blood cells) recognise harmful substances and destroy them.
- Distributes fluid in the body – lymphatic vessels drain approximately 3 litres of excess tissue fluid daily from tissue spaces.
- Transport of fats – carbohydrates and protein are passed from the small intestine directly into the bloodstream. However, fats are passed from the small intestine into lymphatic vessels called lacteals before eventually passing into the bloodstream. It is uncertain why fats are absorbed via the lymphatic system.

Lymph vessels

Lymph travels around the body in one direction only, towards the heart. It is carried in vessels that begin as lymphatic capillaries. Lymph capillaries are blind-ended tubes, situated between cells, and are found throughout the body. The walls of lymphatic capillaries are structured in such a way that tissue fluid can pass into them but not out of them.

The lymphatic system does not have a pump like the heart, but like the veins it relies on the movement of the body and contraction of the skeletal muscles. The squeezing action of the muscles forces the lymph along its vessels. Involuntary actions such as breathing and the heartbeat also help the movement of lymph through the vessels.

Effects of massage on the skin

The circulation is improved and so fresh blood brings nutrients to the sebaceous glands; therefore sebum production is increased. More sebum helps to make the skin soft and supple.

The sweat glands become more active and so more sweat is excreted. Toxins such as urea and other waste products are eliminated from the body in this way.

Massage also causes the top layer of dead skin cells to be shed (desquamation), which improves the condition of the skin, giving it a healthy glow.

The sensory nerve endings can either be soothed or stimulated, depending on the massage movements used.

When massage and essential oils are used together the skin's health and appearance can be greatly improved.

Bones of the head and neck

- Frontal bone – one frontal bone forms the forehead.
- Parietal bone – two parietal bones form the sides and the top of the skull.
- Temporal bone – two temporal bones are found at the sides of the skull under the parietals.
- Occipital bone – one occipital bone forms the back of the skull.
- Ethmoid bone – one ethmoid bone helps to form the eye socket and nasal cavities.
- Sphenoid bone – one sphenoid bone helps to form the base of the skull.
- Cervical spine – consists of seven vertebrae.

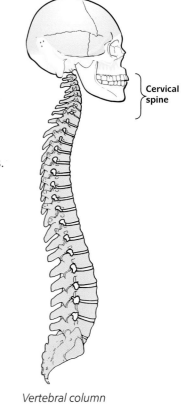

Vertebral column

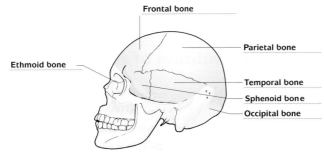

Bones of the skull

Muscles of the head and neck

MUSCLE	POSITION	ACTION
Frontalis	Across the forehead	Draws scalp forward and raises eyebrows
Temporalis	Extends from the temple region to the upper jaw bone	Raises the lower jaw and draws it backwards, as in chewing
Sterno-cleidomastoid	Runs from the top of the sternum to the clavicle and temporal bones	Both together bend head forward; one muscle only rotates the head and draws it towards the opposite shoulder
Platysma	Extends from the lower jaw to the chest and covers the front of the neck	Depresses lower jaw and draws lower lip outwards and draws up the skin of the chest
Occipitalis	At the back of the head	Draws the scalp backwards

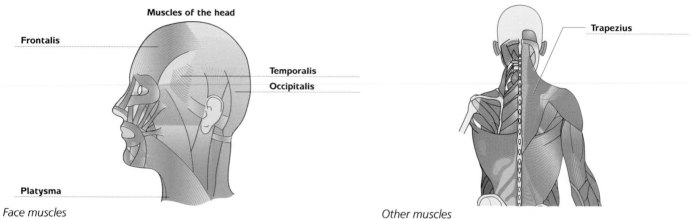

Face muscles

Other muscles

MUSCLE	POSITION	ORIGIN	INSERTION	ACTION
Trapezius	Forms a large, kite-shaped muscle across the top of the back and the neck	Occipital bone and vertebrae	Scapula and clavicle	Lifts the clavicle, as in shrugging and also draws the head backwards

The frontalis is joined to the occipitalis muscle by a strong, flat, broad tendon called the epicranial aponeurosis, which acts as a hat, covering the scalp.

Factors affecting the condition of the skin

Re-read the section in Chapter 1 that deals with the condition of the hair. In this section we will look at the factors affecting the condition of the skin.

Ageing of the skin may occur naturally or it may prematurely age because of various factors, including heredity, environment (perhaps work outside in all weathers), inadequate diet, smoking or ill health.

- Diet – a good, well-balanced diet can help maintain good skin and hair condition. Deficiencies of certain vitamins such as vitamin A, C and B3 can lead to dry skin conditions and dermatitis.

- Alcohol – dehydrates the skin and robs the body of vitamins B and C.

- Caffeine – in large quantities can interfere with the absorption of vitamins and minerals, which can result in unhealthy skin.

- Sunlight – dehydrates the skin causing skin damage, interferes with the structure of collagen and elastin fibres, causing premature ageing of the skin.

- Smoking – slows down blood circulation, destroys vitamin C and interferes with the production of collagen. People who have smoked for a long time will generally look 10 years older than people of the same age.

- Medication – certain medications taken by mouth can lead to skin dehydration, fluid retention or swelling of the tissues – steroids are an example.

- Hydrocortisone creams – applied externally and used to treat skin conditions such as psoriasis and dermatitis. The cream should be used for short lengths of time and in small quantities otherwise thinning of the skin may result.

- Antibiotics – can cause temporary drying of the skin, although it will improve after the course of drugs has finished.

- Taking the contraceptive pill – can cause a condition known as chloasma, where areas of increased pigmentation occur on the skin, usually on the face.

- Central heating, air conditioning and pollution – all dehydrate the skin. Capillaries contract and dilate to adapt to a particular temperature. Constant contracting and dilating will cause thread veins commonly seen on the cheeks and nose.

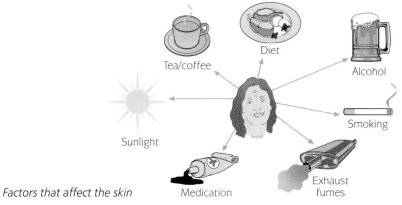

Factors that affect the skin

Contraindications to massage

Scalp massage is a very safe treatment. However, there are certain conditions that the therapist should be aware of which may prevent treatment being carried out or may require the advice of a doctor.

Contraindications or cases where you should never massage the scalp include:

- any recent head or neck injury
- severe bruising, cuts or abrasions in the treatment area
- epilepsy
- recent haemorrhage
- high blood pressure
- low blood pressure
- migraine
- history of thrombosis
- diabetes
- spastic conditions
- dysfunction of the nervous system
- skin disorders/scalp infections
- recent operations.

These are discussed in more detail below.

Any recent head or neck injury

If a client is suffering with concussion or has a neck injury such as whiplash, it is wise not to give treatment as not only could it be uncomfortable for the client but you could worsen the condition.

If the injury is minor, such as a pulled muscle in the neck or shoulders, gentle massage may benefit the client.

Severe bruising, cuts of abrasions in the treatment area

Bruises, cuts and abrasions are localised contraindications. This means that massage can be carried out around them, but if bruising or cuts are severe it may be wise to ask the client to return after the affected area has healed. If there is slight bleeding, ensure that a plaster covers the affected area and that you do not touch it (to prevent cross-infection).

Epilepsy

Epilepsy is a disorder of the brain in which the patient suffers fits (convulsions). The convulsions are due to a surge of overactivity in the brain's electrical system. Usually there is no obvious cause; however, in some case the fits are due to scars on the brain from surgery or injury. Some sufferers find that flickering fluorescent lights or television screens can spark off a fit. The advice of a doctor should be sought before treatment is carried out.

Recent haemorrhage

'Haemorrhage' is the term for excessive bleeding, which can be internal or external. It is advisable not to give treatment to someone who has had a recent haemorrhage because the massage may cause further bleeding.

High blood pressure

High blood pressure (hypertension) is when the blood pressure is consistently above normal. It can lead to strokes and heart attacks as the heart has to work harder to force blood through the system. High blood pressure can be caused by smoking, obesity, lack of exercise, eating too much salt, stress, too much alcohol, the contraceptive pill, pregnancy and hereditary factors.

Massage increases the blood circulation, thus possibly increasing the blood pressure, but as vasodilation (widening of the blood vessels) also occurs there could be a side-effect to massage of lowering the blood pressure, especially after a while. These effects probably counterbalance each other. Massage treatment is also relaxing, so can be of benefit to people with high blood pressure that has been brought on by stress. However, abnormal blood pressure is an important contraindication and it is advisable to seek the advice of the client's doctor.

Low blood pressure

Low blood pressure (hypotension) is when the blood pressure is below normal for a substantial time. Blood pressure must be sufficient to pump blood to the brain when the body is in the upright position. If it is not then the person will feel faint. It is advisable to seek the advice of a doctor before treatment of someone with low blood pressure.

Migraine

Migraines are severe headaches which can last from a couple of hours to a couple of days. The headache is often on one side of the head and other symptoms include nausea, vomiting and sensitivity to light.

It is uncertain what causes migraines, but during an attack the blood vessels in the brain are dilated. Stress and certain foods such as cheese and chocolate may be triggers.

It is extremely unlikely that someone would ask for scalp massage treatment while suffering a migraine.

History of thrombosis or embolism

Thrombosis is the clotting of blood that is stationary within an artery or vein. It is dangerous as it may constrict or cut off the flow of blood. If massage is carried out there is a risk that the clot may be moved or broken up and taken to the heart, lungs or brain, which could prove fatal.

Embolism is the blockage of an artery with a clot of material that is contained within the bloodstream. The clot can be made up of a number of things, including air, fat, bone marrow or even a piece broken off a thrombosis. It circulates in the bloodstream until it becomes wedged somewhere in a blood vessel and blocks the flow of blood. Such a blockage may be extremely harmful. Do not treat clients with thrombosis or embolism and, if the client has a history of either of these conditions, obtain their doctor's advice.

Diabetes

Diabetes mellitus results from too little output of insulin from a gland called the pancreas. Insulin is needed to allow glucose (sugar) into the body's cells so the body can use it to make energy. Lack of insulin causes the sugar to build up in the blood instead. Some symptoms indicating diabetes include tiredness, weight loss, excessive thirst and excessive urination.

People with poorly controlled diabetes may have related conditions such as high blood pressure, hardened arteries, altered sensations in limbs such as numbness, eyesight problems, poor healing of the skin and wasting of the tissues, including the skin, which may be paper-thin. It is advisable to seek the advice of their doctor before treatment.

Spastic conditions
When the muscles are in spasm – in a state of contraction – massage could be uncomfortable for the client.

Dysfunction of the nervous system
Dysfunctions of the nervous system include conditions such as multiple sclerosis, cerebral palsy, Parkinson's disease and motor neurone disease. The doctor's advice should be sought prior to treatment.

Skin disorders/scalp infections
Treatment can be given if the skin disorder or scalp infection is not infectious, there is no bleeding or weeping and it would not cause discomfort when massaged. Otherwise the client should return when the condition has cleared.

Recent operations
If the client has had any recent operations to the area you intend to treat, especially within the last six months, it is wise not to carry out the massage treatment. If the operation is minor, the doctor's advice can be sought.

Other contraindications to massage
Never massage the scalp:

- when there are any infections (e.g. ringworm) or infestations (e.g. head lice) present
- if there are any cuts or abrasions on the scalp
- if the scalp is inflamed or sore to touch
- if the client has any medical problems, even a high temperature, as with colds or flu.

Massage movements

Effleurage
This is a stroking movement, which begins and ends the massage procedure. With your fingers spread slightly apart and starting at the front hairline, apply an even pressure as you slowly slide your fingers through the hair down to the nape in a continuous movement. You should cover most parts of the scalp with your fingers, so that when you repeat the movement several times the client starts to relax.

Petrissage
Petrissage is a deeper, kneading movement, using the pads of the fingers. It stimulates the muscles and nerves, improving the blood circulation. Move your finger pads in a circular direction, picking up and kneading the scalp.

People with a lot of thick hair often have a 'mobile' scalp, which is easy to knead, but others with fine, thin hair may have a tight scalp, which is more difficult to work with. Take care not to pull fine, sparse hair.

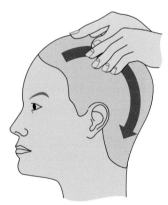

Effleurage

Always ask the client if your massage is comfortable. If you are unsure about the amount of pressure to use, try out the massage on your own scalp first.

During petrissage, start at the front hairline, knead around the top of the head, then gradually work towards the nape area. This massage may last for 5–10 minutes.

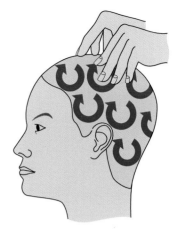
Petrissage

Friction
This is a light, rubbing movement using the finger pads. It is stimulating rather than relaxing and it is not always carried out. It is only done for a few minutes, again working from front to back.

Tapotement
These movements are described as tapping or hacking with the fingertips or the sides of the hands. All tapotement movements are stimulating and so are rarely used in a relaxing type of massage.

Vibrations
Vibrations through the hands or fingers of one hand produce tremors in the tissues, stimulating sluggish lymphatic drainage and relieving fatigue and pain.

High-frequency machines
A **high-frequency machine** uses an alternating electric current to stimulate the blood flow to the scalp increasing the flow of nutrients and oxygen to the hair follicles encouraging hair growth. This treatment can benefit cases of avoidable hair loss.

High-frequency treatments can be used directly on the scalp or indirectly using a saturator.

There are two attachments or electrodes for use with this type of machine. A flat, round bulb is for use on patches of bare skin such as alopecia and is moved in circles over the affected area. A glass rake is used on a full head of hair or thinning hair. The operator literally rakes the hair from the hairline to the crown.

Whether using the direct method where the current flows directly to the client's scalp or the indirect method where the client holds a metal bar with an insulated handle and the current passes through the client's body, the operator must start the frequency on zero, increasing within the comfort zone of the client and finishing on zero to prevent sparking and keeping the electrode in contact with the client throughout the process.

Health and safety
Before using either of these methods the operator must check the machine for any faults, loose wires or flexes. Ask the client to remove all jewellery, and the client's hair must be dry.

TO DO
Read the instructions for your salon's high-frequency machine.

Using heat to assist the penetration of conditioners

Applying heat to oils, conditioning creams and deep-acting conditioners will encourage them to penetrate further into the hair.

Steamers

These look like hand hairdryers but must be warmed up before use. They produce moist heat through the evaporation of distilled water (tap water would make them fur up – like a kettle). The steam swells the hair and raises the cuticle scales so that the product can penetrate more thoroughly. Steamers are particularly useful for African Caribbean hair.

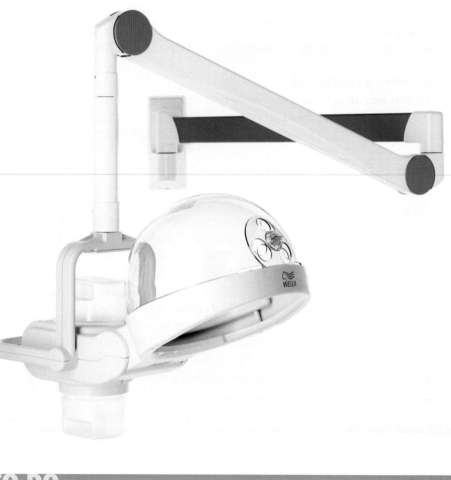

Steamers

Wella

TO DO

Read the section in Chapter 3 on the safe use of electrical equipment.

Hood dryers

These also produce a dry heat. Hot, dry air circulates to dry the hair. A plastic cap is placed over the hair and product before use. Remember to warm the **hood dryer** first by turning it on for several minutes before the client is ready to use it.

Accelerators

Accelerators produce a radiant dry heat, which helps penetration. A plastic cap may need to be used to stop the product from drying out.

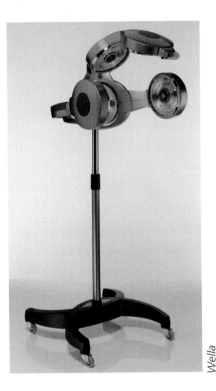

Wella

An accelerator

Record cards

Always keep record cards of the client's treatments. Here is an example.

TREATMENT RECORD CARD							
Name							
Address							
					Tel. no.		
Date	Hair condition	Scalp condition	Product used	Equipment used	Time	Other details	Stylist

Treatment record card

The client could have both hair problems (e.g. over-processed, dry ends) and scalp problems (e.g. a naturally greasy scalp) at the same time, and this should be evident from their record card. If this is the case, deal with the worst problem first, then, when this has been corrected, start to treat the second problem.

1 Briefly describe how the structure of hair relates to conditioning treatments.

2 What is the name of the gland that can cause seborrhoea?

3 Which part of the scalp causes pityriasis capitis?

4 Why is it sometimes beneficial to apply conditioners before chemical processing and at other times after chemical processing?

5 What is the name of the substance that conditions hair naturally?

6 Name the differences between each massage technique.

7 Describe the benefits of scalp massage.

8 State when scalp massage should not be used.

9 Describe why the pH of various products is important to both hair condition and subsequent salon services.

10 Describe how the skin helps to maintain body temperature.

11 List the seven bones of the head and neck.

12 List the five main muscles of the head and neck.

13 Describe the factors that may affect the condition of the skin.

14 When would the high-frequency machine be of use?

15 Why are steamers and hood dryers used during conditioning treatments?

Chapter 6 Blow drying, setting and dressing

After working through this chapter you will be able to:

- Maintain effective and safe methods of working
- Understand hair growth patterns
- Style hair using basic techniques
- Dry and finish hair for men
- Dress and finish hair using the correct tools and products
- Dress long hair using dexterity and manipulation
- Style hair using basic plaiting and added hair
- Understand the different types of added hair available
- Understand the contraindications of added hair and prolonged plaiting
- Prepare the hair to be added
- Produce plaited styles with added hair.

This chapter covers the following NVQ Level 2 units:
Style Dress and Finish Hair Using Basic Techniques
Dry Hair into Shape for Men
Style Hair using Basic Plaiting Techniques and Added Hair

Blow drying

Hair types and textures

You will need to understand the different hair types (European, African Caribbean or Asian) and textures (fine or coarse), to know what tools (e.g. size of brush), techniques (e.g. blow dry, **scrunch dry**) and products (e.g. blow dry lotion, mousse or gel) to use.

Hair growth patterns

TO DO

Re-read the section in Chapter 1 on hair growth patterns.

Natural growth patterns and root movement are just as important when blow drying as when cutting. If you blow dry with the natural fall (the way the hair falls on its own), the style will last longer and the client will find it easier to manage.

TO DO

Re-read the section in Chapter 1 on designing a hairstyle to suit your client.

TEST YOUR KNOWLEDGE

1 Why is it important to keep your work area clean and tidy and avoid cross-infections and infestations?

2 Describe the ways in which the following critical factors can influence your choice of style:

- hair elasticity
- hair texture
- hair cut
- head and face shape
- hair growth patterns.

Why the shape of hair can change through blow drying

All hair is elastic and stretchy. It becomes more elastic when it is thoroughly wet, when it can stretch up to half its length again.

TO DO

Re-read the section in Chapter 1 on hair structure.

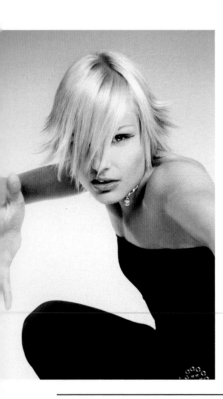

Wet hair stretches because the temporary bonds (the hydrogen bonds and salt links) that join the polypeptide chains in the cortex are broken. However, they quickly rejoin into a new shape when you blow dry the hair.

You can blow dry:

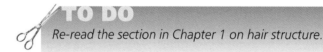

curly and wavy hair ⟶ straight

and

straight hair ⟶ wavy

by breaking the temporary bonds, stretching the hair with a brush and then drying it.

Hair in its natural state – whether curly, wavy or straight – is described as being in an **alpha keratin** state. When the hair is wetted, stretched into a new shape and then dried, it is in a **beta keratin** state.

Once the hair is dampened again – by shampooing or just by being caught out in the rain – then it will go back to its natural state (curly, wavy or straight) and be in the alpha keratin state again.

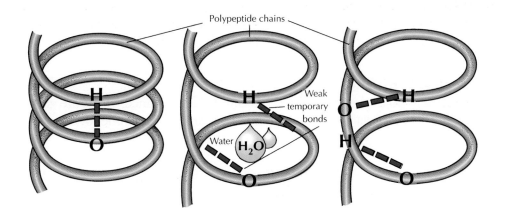

Alpha and beta keratin

Blow drying aids and products

Your hair goes flat when the weather is damp and miserable because hair is hygroscopic. This means it absorbs moisture from the atmosphere (humidity) and the stretched (beta keratin) blow dried shape reverts to its natural (alpha keratin) shape.

To stop this from happening, and to make the blow dry last longer, blow dry lotion, mousse or gel is used. These work in the same way as hairspray, in that they coat the hair with a very fine film of plastic to stop the hair absorbing moisture. These plastic resins help to protect the hair from heat and damage during blow drying.

It is important to use products intended for blow drying – setting lotions will make the hair too sticky to work with.

Always apply blow dry aids to towel-dried hair, because if the hair is too wet the product will be diluted. Check the manufacturer's instructions, but you will find that you should apply most gels and mousses by placing them in the centre of your palm and then spreading them evenly over the hair with your fingers. Blow dry lotions must be sprinkled evenly over the hair.

TO DO

The client will have already been gowned up for shampooing. Check with your supervisor if a special-colour towel is needed while applying colour products which could stain light-coloured towels.

Some blow dry products contain colours, such as silver, ash or copper, which wash out of the hair. Only use these with the help of your supervisor or once you have learned about colouring (this is described in Chapter 10) – you may find the hair turns out the colour of a carrot!

Finally, after blow drying you can use a hairspray for extra hold, or spray-on shine or wax for a glossy finish.

TO DO

Find out which blow dry products in your salon are suitable for:

- *fine hair*
- *coarse hair*
- *curly hair*
- *straight hair*
- *a soft or casual look*
- *a firm hold*
- *a wild, full look.*

Tools and equipment for blow drying

Blow drying brushes

Flat or paddle brushes

Used to dry and polish for sleek styles, but can also add bounce. These are good for smooth finishes, especially for bob haircuts. They are not recommended for very curly results.

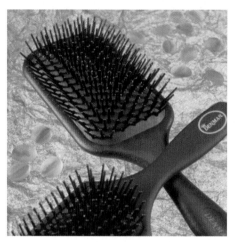

Flat/paddle brush

Vent brushes

The vented holes allow the **air flow** from the hairdryer to pass through, speeding up the drying process by heating the hair, while the short filaments break up the hair so that it lies as if fingers have been drawn through it creating casual styles. Good for brushing out sets and hairstyles to create natural, casual looks with a soft 'broken' effect. They can become tangled in the hair.

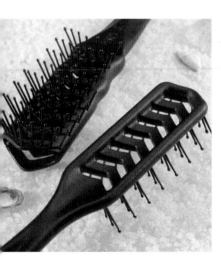

Vent brush

Circular or round brushes

Used to produce a curl or wave movement by slowly rotating the hair around the brush while blow drying the hair. The smaller the brush the tighter the curl. Suitable for most hair lengths except very long hair, which is not layered. Circular brushes can easily tangle in the hair if the hair is fine or long. The diameter of the brush determines the degree and tightness of the curl. Circular brushes are also good for adding bounce and curl to the points of one-length styles. The smaller barrel sizes are ideal for shorter length styling and those hard-to-reach areas such as around the ears.

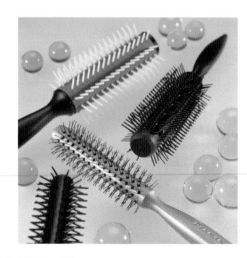

Circular/round brush

Half twist or half round Denman brushes

These are perfect for brushing out a roller set. The maximum effect is achieved by placing the brush into the hairline and rotating the brush, in a half twist movement, by drawing it through the hair.

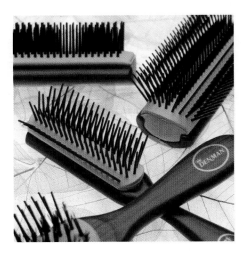

Half twist/half round Denman brushes

Bristle or Denman brushes

A very popular brush used to smooth hair and give lift to simple shapes, such as the bob. These smooth the hair, polishing and helping create gloss finishes.

The more tightly packed soft bristles are suited for finer hair.

Hard-bristle brushes work best on thicker, coarser hair types.

Metal/ceramic core brushes

The metal barrel when heated by the dryer acts as a hot brush. It styles the hair quicker by drying and styling. Gives very good curl movement.

Finishing brushes

Dense-bristle brushes, can be either soft or stiff and are used to finish styles and brush out sets and for back-brushing.

Metal-bristle brushes should be tipped and coated with tiny balls. The base should be made from flexible rubber.

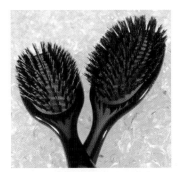

Bristle/Denman brush

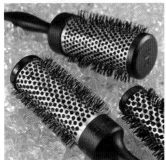

Metal core brush

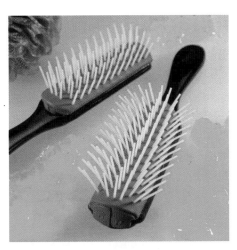

Finishing brush

Combs

Rake combs

These combs are used for disentangling the hair after shampooing. They always have widely spaced teeth, and do not tear or stretch wet hair.

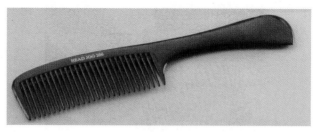

Rake comb

Straight medium-tooth comb/cutting comb

These have two sizes of teeth and are made in various lengths and sizes.
They are mainly used for sectioning the hair before blow drying and while assessing the natural growth patterns and root lift.

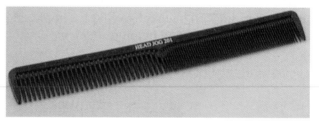

Straight medium-tooth comb

The finer teeth are useful for back-combing. The wider teeth are useful for disentangling hair, finger waving and straightening, while blow drying. If using to straighten hair, the comb must be heat resistant.

Sectioning clips

Sectioning clips or butterfly clamps are needed to hold large sections of hair apart during blow drying.

Electrical appliances

Hand hairdryers

Hand-held dryers/diffusers are a matter of personal choice when drying hair, but consideration should be given to the following:

- choose a reputable manufacturer (both for value and safety)
- consider the weight of the dryer (it can prove important by the end of a day's work)
- if possible, choose one with various heat/speed selections and a 'cold' button if available
- check the guard/vent can be easily removed for cleaning
- check for correct voltage, plugs, wiring, fuses etc.

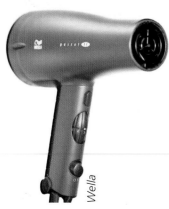

Hairdryer

Wella

- you will want to use **dryer attachments** (see below) for extra effectiveness.

Precautions

- Make sure all plugs are wired correctly.
- Always check the manufacturer's instructions regarding heat settings and speed controls before you start blow drying.
- Make sure that the dryer cable and plug are always safe (look out for frayed wires and loose plug tops).
- Hairdryers have an air intake grill at the back which must be cleaned regularly to remove dust and fluff. If they are not cleaned regularly they may overheat and become dangerous.
- Store electrical tools in accordance with your salon's requirements (e.g. don't allow flexes to trail on the floor, where feet can become caught up in them).

HEALTH MATTERS

Standing all day long

Arms and body

Muscles are used for two kinds of work, dynamic and static. Dynamic work is when the muscles are moving and the blood is pumping through them. Static work is when the muscles are being held in position. The latter can restrict the blood flow, causing waste products to accumulate, and making the muscles tired, tense and stiff. Therefore you should keep your muscles as relaxed as possible by changing the way in which you hold yourself.

For instance, move around your client when you are working on the sides of their hair – don't stand at the back and stretch over or you could strain your back.

It is also useful to learn how to use the hairdryer and brush with either hand, swapping over occasionally. This will help to keep the weight of the dryer balanced by using both arms. Sometimes the lead of the dryer will not reach around the client, so you have to learn to use both hands when using a hairdryer!

Dryer attachments

Nozzles

When these are attached to the hairdryer the air flow is concentrated, which is useful for drying both short hair and small sections of hair.

Diffusers

These have the opposite effect to a nozzle. With diffusers, the air is dispersed over a wider area and the air flow is less forceful. They are often used for drying curly hair.

Nozzle

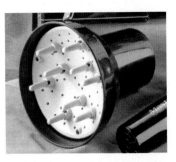

Diffuser

Electric curling tongs or irons

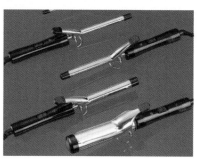

Electric curling irons

Electric tongs are thermally heated equipment, consisting of a metal cylinder barrel, around which hair is wrapped to add curl or wave movement. Diameter sizes of the barrel can range from pencil thin to hairspray can size. They should have more than one heat setting and a clamp that is easy to use.

Tongs can be used to produce a variety of effects, from curls and waves to **ringlets**. They are often used after blow drying to 'firm up' the shape of the curl produced by a circular brush.

The ends of the hair must be wound smoothly around the tongs or you will produce distorted or buckled ends.

All tongs have a thermostat inside them to prevent overheating, but remember that they can still burn. Many also have a flex with a swivel action to prevent the cord from becoming twisted.

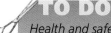

TO DO

Health and safety requirements:
- *Read the Electricity at Work Regulations 1992, including the section on using electrical equipment safely, in Chapter 3, and state your responsibilities.*
- *Make a list of any pieces of electrical equipment in your salon that you think are unsafe. Check it with your supervisor.*

Hot brushes

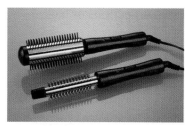

Hot brush

Hot brushes are easier to use than tongs but you cannot achieve quite as many different effects (such as ringlets) with them. Again, they have a thermostat inside them and the flex may have a swivel action.

Hot brushes work in the same way as tongs but the teeth or bristles help to grip the hair. They can be easier to work with than tongs, but you must take clean sections or they can become tangled in the hair.

- *Find out all the different tools and equipment available for drying hair in your salon.*
- *Check the answers with your supervisor.*

Straighteners and crimping irons

Straightening irons and crimping irons are thermally heated plates that are either smooth, to produce a straight finish, or textured to produce wave/crimp movement. Some irons are reversible to create either textured hair or straight hairstyles.

Crimping irons

Textured plates produce a pattern of straight-line crimps on straight hair. They create volume, making the hair appear thicker, and are useful for long hair.

To use the crimpers, take neat sections of the hair no wider than the metal plates of the crimpers and close the iron for 2–5 seconds on the hair. Release, then move down to the next part of the straight hair, press again and release. Continue until all the hair is crimped.

Straightening irons

These have smooth plates to produce extra straight, flat hair and are ideal for making dense hair appear less bulky.

These electrical hair straighteners sometimes have ceramic plates which are less damaging on the hair.

Small straightening tongs are used to smooth short hair or add soft wave movement to hair ends.

REMEMBER

Tongs, hot brushes and crimping irons should be cleaned with cotton wool or disinfectant spray or wipes – never immersed in water.

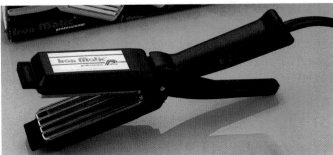

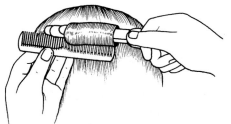

Straightening irons

Precautions for using tongs, hot brushes, straighteners and crimping irons

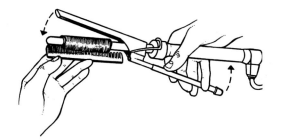

Using tongs etc.

- Always pick them up by their handles.
- Always place a comb between hot tongs and the client's scalp when you are working near the scalp.
- Always use the stand or rest attached to the tongs to prevent work surfaces from becoming scorched and plastic surfaces (such as equipment trolleys) from melting.
- Never put hot tongs into your tool bag. Allow them to cool first.
- Remember to switch off the tongs as soon as you have finished using them – it helps to prevent accidents.
- Light-coloured hair can be discoloured and scorched by the tongs, so do not have them too hot or use them for too long on the hair.
- All flexes can become twisted and the insulation can gradually wear away, making the tools dangerous. Flexes must be checked regularly.

Advice to clients using heated styling equipment at home
- Check the appliances for safety (see page 3).
- Use a hairdryer nozzle for drying short and small sections of hair.
- Use a hairdryer diffuser for drying curly hair.
- Don't have the tongs too hot.
- Don't allow tongs to rest for too long on the hair.
- Make sure the hair ends are wound smoothly around the tongs.
- Take great care using hot brushes on long hair – they can easily become entangled and difficult to remove.
- Place a comb underneath the tongs when working near the skin or scalp.
- Hair 'bubbling': many home-use heated appliances must be used with 80 per cent dry hair. If the hair is too wet the tools (which operate at 120–180°C) will boil the water in the hair (water boils at 100°C). Bubbles will form inside the hair shaft and the hair will eventually break off at, or somewhere near, the bubble.

Using mirrors when blow drying

During blow drying, as with combing out and finishing the style, you need to look continually in the mirror to check the **balance** of the hairstyle. You must make sure it is not lopsided and that there are no large breaks or holes in the dressing.

Technical points to remember when blow drying and styling hair

- Confirm the desired result with your client, using visual aids such as photographs if necessary.
- Always towel dry the hair first (except for very curly, very fine or very short hair) to save drying time. Excess moisture should be towel blotted from the hair after shampooing. When towel drying refrain from rubbing against the hair as damage to the cuticle scales can occur, causing tangles. Instead blot the hair by gently squeezing.
- The choice of product should be applied evenly to the hair following the manufacturer's instructions. Care should be taken to avoid the product coming into contact with the client's eyes and skin.

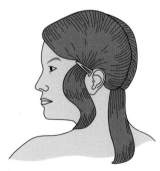

Hair sectioned for blow drying

- Remember that a style always lasts longer if it follows the **natural movement** of the hair.
- The appropriate brush or brushes should be selected for the required style.
- Comb the hair to remove any tangles. Follow the direction of the finished style, then section according to the size of the brush you have chosen. Ensure that dry sections do not mix with wet sections.
- Sections should be neat and clean.
- The dryer should be set at the correct heat and speed.
- The stream of air should follow the brush at the correct distance from the strand.
- The filter end must be kept clean as blockage will prevent air passing through freely and can cause the dryer to overheat and become dangerous to use.
- Make sure each section is thoroughly dry before you take the next section.
- The root area is normally dried first – to increase volume the outflow should be directed towards the roots.

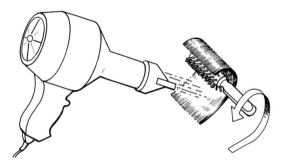

Drying into the roots to increase volume

- Always work from roots to points, keeping the cuticle scale flat.
- Keep the dryer moving to prevent burning the hair or the scalp. If the dryer is too hot the hair cuticle may be damaged and the hair could break.
- Always lift the hair while removing the brush to prevent tangling.
- Keep an even tension on the hair but do not overstretch it by pulling too hard.

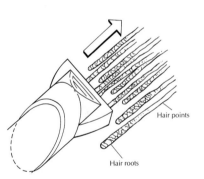

Keeping the cuticle flat

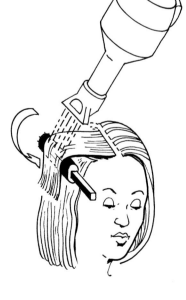

Correct

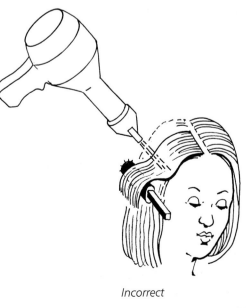

Incorrect

Correct and incorrect blow drying

Common faults when blow drying

- Using clips to hold fragile hair while drying can mark the hair.
- Uneven sectioning can create an uneven finish.
- Over-drying the hair can cause the hair to look dry and dull.
- Under-drying the hair will cause the hair to lose its shape and style quickly.
- Using incorrect brushes and tools can damage the hair shaft.

Men's blow drying

Techniques used on women's hair can also be used on men's hair; the most popular drying techniques are:

- finger drying – suitable for short, spiky, curly or unstructured styles
- blow drying – various brushes can be used. The finished look often has minimum lift and a square finished shape
- **blow waving** – a traditional technique that creates waves in the hair to look like **finger waves**.

Blow waving

This is suitable on short hair with wave movement. It is mostly used in men's hairdressing although it is equally as good for female clients. Blow waving can be difficult to do on sparse hair and should be in the direction of the natural growth patterns on the front hairline. Always use the nozzle attachment to create lifted wave movements, and use the dryer on half speed. Always work with the natural fall.

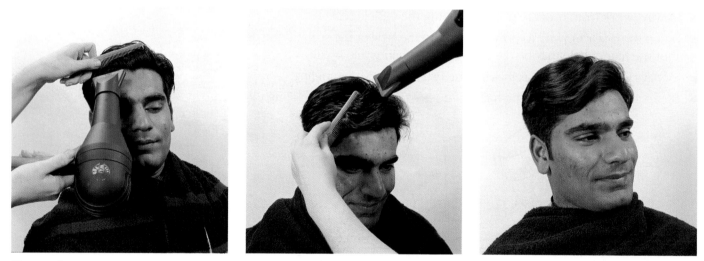

Blow waving

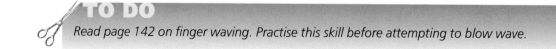

TO DO

Read page 142 on finger waving. Practise this skill before attempting to blow wave.

Allow hair to cool completely (cold shots of air from the dryer help), then check it is quite dry. Warm hair can be deceptively damp.

Keep checking the shape of the hairstyle in the mirror, and always show your client the back.

DRYING METHOD	EFFECT	SUITABILITY
Flat brush	Used for a smooth finish, e.g. a 'bob'	Hair requiring only a slight curve or straight finish; curl cannot be achieved
Vent brush	Produces a soft, casual, 'broken up' effect	Good for a quick casual result, but not very suitable for curling
Circular brush	Good for producing a curled effect; the the smaller the brush the tighter the finished curl	Large circular brushes are used to curl the ends of long hair. Small brushes give tight curls. Any circular brush tangles easily in the hair
Finger drying	Produces a very natural, casual soft finish. You can also use the palm of your hand to rotate the roots and create lift	Best used for 'fashion' looks. If the client bends forwards and the hair is dried from underneath more lift is achieved at the roots
Natural drying (diffuser, accelerator, infrared, roller ball)	Produces a natural, casual look similar to the shape of the hair when wet	Ideal for drying permed or naturally curly hair, as the hair is not disturbed when drying
Scrunch drying	Produces a rough wave/curl finish with lots of movement	Works best on medium-length, layered hair with some wave and movement
Blow waving	Produces lifted wave movement	For a natural, soft fullness. Often used for drying men's hair, particularly at the front hairline

TO DO

Check with your supervisor how long it should take you to either blow dry or set:

- *short, layered hair*
- *short, one-length hair*
- *long, layered hair*
- *long, one-length hair.*

Then time yourself doing each.

HEALTH MATTERS

Styling

When styling, it is as important to work at the correct height of the client (by adjusting the chair height or by bending your knees) as it is when cutting.

Are your shoes comfortable? Shoes that pinch and are too tight will increase strain, and ones with heels that are too high will cause undue back stress and may make you too tall for the client's height in the chair.

Try to take little breaks when working in order to rest your arms and hands. This is easily done by stopping to explain to your client how to maintain their style or which products (shampoos, conditioners, styling products or hairsprays) they could use at home.

Styling and finishing products

Products used in styling hair fall into two separate categories. There are styling products and finishing products.

Styling products

Blow drying lotions

Generally similar to setting lotions, these contain higher amounts of alcohol to dry the hair quicker and lower amounts of plasticisers to enable the hair to be moulded slower. They are formulated to protect the hair from heat-styling equipment and to help to produce a shine, particularly on straight hair.

Gels

Gels come in various strengths; these can give the strongest hold and shine. They are good for curly and wavy hair definition. They are used for controlling **frizz** and static, defining the line, slicking hair back and moulding and sculpting.

Apply to towel-dry damp or dry hair. Some also help straighten hair by making the hair slippery in texture so blow drying is easier, and gel also flattens the hair. They are excellent for very curly hair in emphasising the individual curls.

Choose formulas that can be brushed out easily without leaving a powdery residue. Gels can also be used as a finishing product.

Groom

Including silicones, these products are applied to damp hair to reduce volume, define texture and smooth sections of hair.

Mousses

Mousses are designed to give a more definite, texturised look to hairstyles, together with added body. They hold styles in place longer.

Sprays

Sprays include styling and volumising, holding and finishing, and mousses. These are body-building products to be used on towel-dried damp hair prior to drying into style.

Sprays can add body and can help define curls and waves and support roots.

Finishing products

These products are applied to previously dried hair to add a 'finished' look to it.

Activators and serums

Activators are types of oil sprays and are used on permed or naturally curly hair to maintain the curl. They must be used sparingly by spray misting over the hair or by applying them to the palms of the hands, rubbing the hands together and then smoothing on the hair.

Serums, which are high-density silicone fluids, are particularly good on dry hair to hold splayed ends together and reduce a ragged appearance.

Brilliantines

There are two types of brilliantines: liquid, which is mineral oil based with perfume and colour; and cream, which is mineral oil mixed with wax and perfume. These add shine to the hair and can added textured definition. They are used mainly within men's hairdressing.

Clays and crèmes

Crèmes add shine and gloss, whereas clays give a matte finish. These add texture and some holding power, keeping the hair in style while giving flexibility.

Dressing creams and pomades

These products have the same uses as gels and waxes but are gentler on the hair. They add shine, retain moisture and help to control the hair. Some may penetrate the hair, helping to 'bind' any damaged areas and protecting the hair from further damage. Silicone based products should be applied to damp hair using small amounts to prevent overloading the hair. These products also reduce tangling and frizzing.

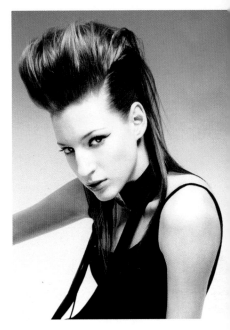

Frictions

Frictions contain perfumed alcohol, which evaporates when massaged. They are used to stimulate the scalp while leaving a scent.

Hair fixing sprays

Fixing sprays contain **synthetic** plastic polymers (polyvinyl pyrrolidone with polyvinyl acetate) which coat the hair with a plastic film without 'gluing' large surface areas of hair together; these also allow the hair to be re-combed with ease. They are suitable for casual styles, allowing clients to comb and rearrange their hair between salon visits without ruining the style.

Hairspray

Hairsprays are normally used when the finished look is to the client's satisfaction. They keep the hair in the desired shape and often contain ingredients to enhance the shine. They must be sprayed 30 cm away from the hair – too close and they will clog the hair and cause a build-up.

Lacquer may contain shellac, which is dissolved in alcohol. When this is sprayed on the hair, the alcohol evaporates, leaving the hair coated in resin. This is suitable for styles that need a lot of support with the minimum of re-combing. Lanolin is sometimes added to enable the spray to be more pliable, as the finished results may be very stiff.

Moisturisers

Moisturisers are used to maintain hair in a shiny, moist condition. They are good for split ends, detangling and to temporarily repair damaged hair. They close the cuticle scales, thus reducing **static electricity**. Fine hair should be lightly moisturised as when the cuticle scales are open the hair has more width and volume. Denser or coarse hair requires heavier formulations to soften and add weight to the hair. Available in gel, cream and spray form. They can be applied to specific areas of the hair shaft and do not have to be applied to the whole head. Use sparingly to avoid build-up.

Wax

Wax is ideal to use on very curly hair and can also be used to dress out a very dramatic look on straight hair.

TEST YOUR KNOWLEDGE

1 Make a list of three different textures and types of hair.
2 Why do you have to consider hair growth patterns when blow drying?
3 State two differences between the properties of wet and dry hair.
4 Describe the effects of humidity on dried hair.
5 Name three different blow drying effects.
6 Describe the tools, equipment and products you would use to achieve these effects.
7 Which government Act relates to the use of electrical drying equipment? Briefly describe its contents.
8 Name the government Act that relates to finishing products. Describe how these products may be hazardous.

African Caribbean hair

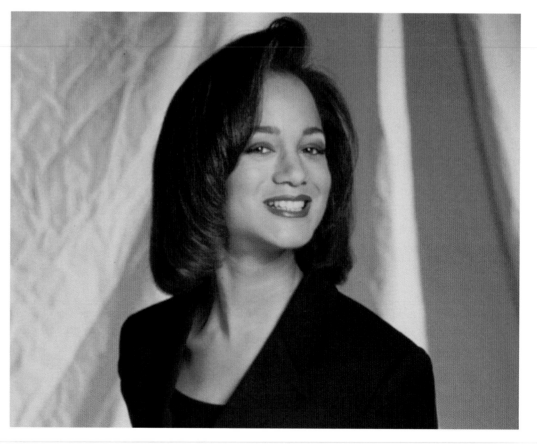

Temporarily straightened African Caribbean hair

REMEMBER

Hair pressing or thermal hair straightening is a temporary process. It breaks the hydrogen bonds by using heat and tension, working in the same way as electric tongs, hot brushes and crimping irons.

African Caribbean hair does not blow dry well unless it has been temporarily straightened by soft pressing or by using a wide-toothed comb **hand-held dryer** attachment. Once the hair is straight it can be moulded into shape with the dryer and circular brushes.

Pressing combs

Regular or non-electric combs

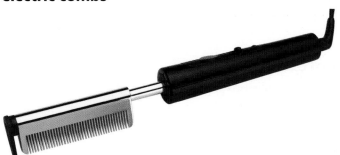

Electric pressing comb

These combs are made of steel or brass and the handle is made of wood. They are heated by small electric heaters or gas stoves. Eight sizes are available, the space between the teeth varying – small teeth are used for fine hair, large teeth for coarse hair.

Thermostatically controlled combs
These have a set working temperature.

Soft pressing

Always check the scalp for soreness (from chemical treatments) or scratches (from previous pressing or styling) before proceeding. Do not continue if you find a problem, but recommend conditioning treatments.

Using this method 70 per cent of the curl can be removed.

The technique
- Shampoo, condition and dry the hair.
- Apply a suitable pressing oil, pomade or cream to the hair and scalp to protect against scorching and to add sheen.
- Take sections of 1.25 cm, starting at the back and holding the hair at 90 degrees to the head. Check the heat of the comb, then insert it 1.25 cm from the scalp.

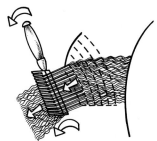

Inserting a pressing comb

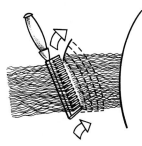

Pulling the hair straight using the back of a pressing comb

- Slide the comb down the hair **mesh**, turning it over so that the back of the comb creates tension and straightens the hair.
- Comb each mesh of hair two or three times and gradually work towards the front.
- Once complete, apply a dressing cream, brush it through and style with curling tongs.

Hard pressing

This method removes almost all of the curl but is more damaging to the hair than soft pressing. Simply repeat the soft pressing method or straighten the hair again with **marcel waving** irons. These non-electric irons are slid down the hair mesh, pulling it straight.

Thermal pressing

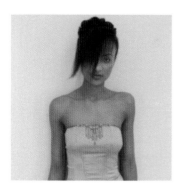

- This process is totally unsuitable for Caucasian hair.
- It can scorch the hair.
- Scalp burns are possible.
- Sweating or damp air etc. will cause the hair to revert back to its natural state.

Cleaning pressing combs

Always wipe the pressing comb so that it is free from grease and loose hairs after use. Clean combs work better, so use a commercially prepared product regularly to help remove carbon build-up.

TEST YOUR KNOWLEDGE

1 What is the effect of heat on hair?
2 How could incorrect application of heat affect the hair and scalp?

REMEMBER

- Check the heat of the pressing comb on white tissue or a white towel. If it scorches, let the comb cool down.
- Fine, bleached and tinted hair all need a lower comb temperature.
- Don't touch the scalp or skin with the hot comb and don't try to straighten very short hair – you could burn the client.
- Pressing normally lasts about 7–10 days but the hair will become curly again if the atmosphere is damp or the client's head perspires.
- No chemicals are used in these processes, so the hair can undergo pressing once a fortnight without undue damage.

Setting and dressing short and long hair

Setting hair can be just as exciting as blow drying hair: the same set on short, medium or long hair can give you three completely different looks when you brush them through.

Deciding on the style

Never say to the client, 'What colour rollers [i.e. size] do you use?'. You are the professional and should be recommending not only what size of rollers but also what type of style will best suit the client. The dentist does not ask which teeth you would like filled, does he?

Always consider the following points:

- Is the set for any particular occasion?
  Is the set for everyday wear or for a special event such as a party, dinner dance or wedding?
- How curly is the hair?
  Curly hair (naturally curly or permed) may need to be straightened for a wavy look by using large rollers. Straight hair may need smaller rollers to produce a curl.
- How long is the hair?
  The longer the hair, the heavier it becomes, so if a client with long, straight hair wants a curly look you will have to use smaller rollers.
- How thick is the hair?
  Clients with a lot of thick, textured hair will need larger rollers, but those with a small amount of fine hair will need smaller rollers.
- How bouncy is the hair?
  'Bounciness' depends on the amount of elasticity in the hair, and clients with limp, lifeless hair (no elasticity) will need smaller rollers.

TO DO

- Re-read the section in Chapter 1 on designing a hairstyle to suit your client.
- Make a short list of the rules that apply when setting (e.g. a client with a short neck will look better with an upswept, flicked style at the nape).

Hair growth patterns

The client's natural hair fall and movement can easily be seen when the hair is wet.

TO DO

Re-read the section in Chapter 1 on hair growth patterns, then for your next client explain the difference between the natural hair fall (or parting) and the hair growth patterns (front hairline, crown area and nape areas) to your supervisor.

If you set the hair with the natural fall or hair growth pattern then the style will last longer and the client will find it easier to manage.

Why the shape of the hair can change through setting (temporary curling)

Setting (also known as temporary curling), like blow drying, is a temporary process (unlike perming, which is a permanent process). This means that we can change the shape of the hair by making curly hair straight or straight hair curly – and if we do not like the result, we can quickly dampen down the hair and change it.

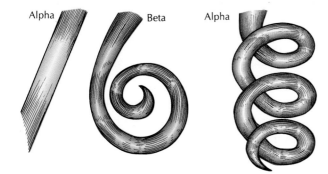

Naturally straight hair becomes curly, changing from alpha to beta keratin

Naturally curly hair becomes straight, changing from alpha to beta keratin

REMEMBER

Hair in its natural unstretched state is known as alpha keratin. Hair in its new, stretched (set) shape is known as beta keratin.

The temporary bonds in the cortex, which are broken during **wet setting** (also known as **cohesive setting**), allow the hair to be stretched even longer (up to half its length again).

TO DO

Re-read the section in Chapter 1 on hair structure. Make a note of which bonds in the cortex are broken during setting and blow drying, and the name of the protein in hair.

Setting aids and products

Sets last much longer in dry atmospheres (like the Middle East) than in damp, humid atmospheres (like the UK), where they drop very quickly. This is because hair is

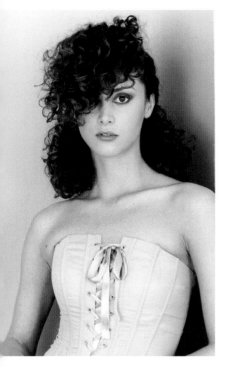

hygroscopic, and the stretched beta keratin (the cohesive set) will gradually return to alpha keratin.

Setting aids such as setting lotion, sculpting lotions, moulding mists or gel coat the hair to keep it from drying out while **winding** and to retain the style for a longer time after the set by stopping moisture from being absorbed into the hair.

Traditional setting lotion ingredients included gum karaya – a soluble vegetable gum mixed with alcohol, perfume and preservative.

Modern setting lotions are based on plasticisers or synthetic plastic polymers, e.g. polyvinyl pyrrolidone. These leave a see-through plastic film on the hair shaft. They can also be pH balanced.

Setting aids are always applied to towel-dried hair; too much water in the hair would dilute the product.

Always check the manufacturer's instructions but, as a rule, most mousses and gels should be placed in the centre of the palm and then spread evenly over the hair with the fingers. Setting lotions must be sprinkled evenly all over the hair.

TO DO

Find out which setting products in your salon are suitable for:
- *fine hair*
- *coarse hair*
- *curly hair*
- *straight hair*
- *use on soft sets*
- *use on tight sets.*

REMEMBER

Excess humidity (a very damp atmosphere) will make sets drop more quickly.

Some setting aids and products contain temporary colours (which wash out of the hair) such as silver, ash, coppers and reds. Use these only under supervision or once you have read Chapter 10. White hair will show the colours much more brightly than you expect.

Hairsprays are used during combing out (or dressing) to control the hair and give more hold and body. They do this in the same way as setting aids, by coating the hair with a very fine film of plastic.

REMEMBER

Always hold hairspray at least 30 cm from the hair while spraying; any closer and the hair becomes too stiff and sticky.

Static electricity

Hair dressings such as spray shines, waxes and creams are used on dry hair to help reduce static electricity, define the shape and finish off the style. They are only used a little at a time because the hair soon becomes over-greasy if too much is used.

TO DO

Find out which products you have in your salon for use as hairsprays (to hold the hair) and which products you have for adding shine.

Tools and equipment for setting and dressing

Brushes

Brushes are used before setting to disentangle the hair before shampooing and during the client consultation, and after setting to remove all the roller marks and to dress the hair.

Flat brushes are normally used with open tufts or bristles which can go through the hair easily without tangling.

Combs

Combs are used to remove tangles (usually when the hair is wet), for parting and sectioning the hair and for combing out or dressing the hair.

Dressing combs

- Used to backcomb and dress out a finished style.
- They have smooth or serrated medium-spaced teeth with prongs on the opposite side (available with two to five plastic or metal prongs).
- The teeth are ideal for backcombing, smoothing and dressing the hair, while the prongs are used to pick up hair strands.

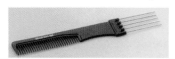

Dressing comb

Tail combs

- **Tail combs** have a plastic or metal tail and usually one size of teeth. They are dual-purpose combs for removing tangles from fine sections and for sectioning the hair.
- They are used for setting, when the tail is useful for tucking the ends of the hair cleanly round the roller.
- The larger teeth are used for disentangling the hair and for forming waves when finger waving, whereas the fine teeth are useful for backcombing.

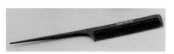

Tail comb

Rake combs

As we have already seen in Chapter 5 on shampooing and conditioning, these combs are useful for disentangling hair after shampooing. They do not tear and stretch the hair because they have wide-spaced teeth.

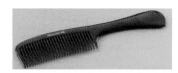

Rake comb

Rollers

There are two common setting rollers.

- Smooth finish rollers, made from plastic, can be used with chemical services, i.e. perm winding. Winding the hair around this type of roller takes practice and pins can be used to hold the roller in place. The smooth finish result makes them ideal for competition work and porous hair.

- Spiked rollers grip the hair more easily, but can be difficult to keep clean and free from hairs. Care must be taken when winding long hair to reduce the chance of hair becoming tangled. Spiked rollers can cause dents or ridges on porous hair.

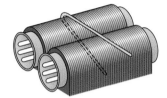

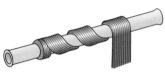

Spiral winding

Rollers secured with straight pin

Most rollers are held in place with either straight pins or setting pins.

Different-sized rollers are available for various effects, and they are often colour coded. Generally, the smaller the roller, the tighter the curl.

Bendable stick rollers
More commonly known as **Molton Browners**. These rubberised tube-shaped rollers are ideal for spiral winding the hair to achieve corkscrew, **spiral curls**.

TO DO

Look at all the sizes of setting rollers in your salon and make a note of the colour code for each size. The smaller the curler the tighter the curl produced.

Pins and clips

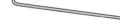

Straight pin

Straight pins
Straight, strong pins are made of metal and must never be used during perming as they will react with the perm lotion and discolour the hair.

They are used to secure rollers during setting and for dressing long hair.

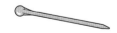

Setting pin

Plastic setting pins
These can also be used to hold rollers in place during setting, but they do tend to distort the hair and leave marks.

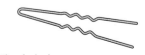

Fine hairpin

Fine hairpins
Hairpins are mainly used during combing out, especially when putting up long hair. They are often available in several shades to match the client's hair colour. They are not very strong and will hold only small amounts of hair.

Hairgrips

Hairgrips, like fine hairpins, are available in a variety of colours to match the client's hair colour, and are mostly used for long hair.

The flat prong is always placed flat to the head, and the ends of both prongs are covered with plastic to prevent them from scratching the client's scalp.

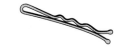

Hairgrip

Double-pronged clips

These can be made of metal or plastic and are usually used for securing **pin curls**.

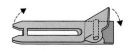

Double-pronged clip

Hairnets

Nylon setting nets are usually triangular in shape and are used to keep rollers and pin curls in place while the client is under the dryer. Ear shields may also be used to protect the client's ears under the hairdryer, but they must be clean and sterile.

Hood dryers

These are used to dry the hair where rollers or pin curls have been used, or for natural drying under a slow speed setting. They may be part of a drying bank, attached to the wall or portable (freestanding) and moved to the dressing position. Always remember to show your client how to use the dryer controls.

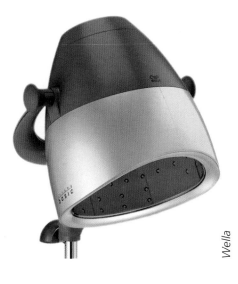

Wella

Hood dryer

Using mirrors when setting

During setting you will need to use your mirror to check that the sections and partings are in the right place. You also need your mirror to check the shape of the hairstyle for balance and to make sure there are no breaks or holes in the finished work.

Setting techniques (cohesive setting)

Cohesive or wet setting involves wetting the hair (shampooing), and towel drying to remove excess moisture. The hair should be kept damp while winding as the 'water breakable' bonds or salt links need to be kept broken to enable the hair to be moulded.

A set will retain its curl or wave movement better and last longer if the hair is damp combed into its natural hair fall and wound tightly.

Setting agents applied can help retain the moisture in the hair to aid winding.

Setting lotions help soften the hair, to mould and keep the hair damp prior to drying. Once dried, setting lotions coat the hair with a fine film that resists moisture and static, preventing 'fly away' hair.

Setting or styling products used prior to drying should be applied to damp hair to prevent dilution and product weakening.

Always apply the recommended amount to prevent flaking by over-application. Decide the style with your client. Then choose the size of rollers and decide whether you need to use any pin curls.

Once the hair is dried and has cooled down, check by unwinding one roller and touching the hair; damp hair will feel cold and will not have firm wave movement. A roller set should be allowed to cool before removing the rollers, otherwise the curl shape may relax slightly, reducing the staying power and causing curl weakening. Also it is sometimes pleasant for the clients to cool themselves down after the time spent under a warm hood dryer!

The final set is called the **pli** (pronounced 'plee').

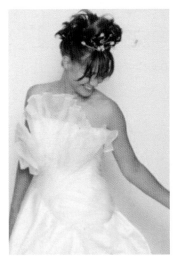

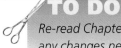

TO DO

Re-read Chapter 1 to find out how to gown and protect your client for setting, including any changes needed for using temporary colours.

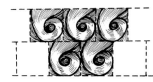

Sections for pin curls

Sectioning

Sectioning allows you to work methodically (step by step) and without getting muddled.

The size and areas of section will depend on what you are doing. For example, pin curls need small, square sections, but rollers need larger, oblong sections.

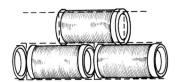

Sections for rollers

To section the hair, comb the hair flat then use your tail comb to draw a clean line with the end of the teeth of the comb along the scalp. The hair should then be parted in two. Hold the hair apart with one hand, then comb the hair down either side to create a clean parting.

REMEMBER

Sections for rollers must have clean lines and be just a little smaller than the roller size.

If you are rollering, place the roller on the hair to measure the width of the section (it should be just shorter than the roller) and make a second parting parallel to the first. To complete the oblong section use the tail end of the comb (without teeth) underneath the roller to complete the third line of the section.

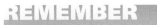

TO DO

Practise making clean, neat sections for rollers. Sections must be good for setting, but perfect for perming (the sections for perming are the same but smaller).

Setting with rollers

Rollers are used to create volume and lift in the finished style.

It is easier to start at the top of the head, but always plan your pli in your mind before starting. Think about which size of rollers will be used on which area of the head and where the pin curls will be placed.

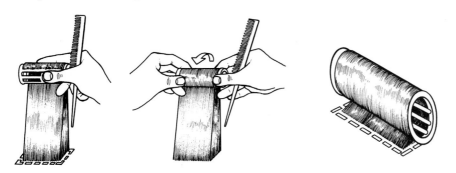

Once the section has been taken, comb the hair smoothly and evenly, without using any undue tension or pulling too much. Take the roller and wind the hair evenly and cleanly down to the scalp so that the roller sits on its base, then secure it with a pin.

Never allow the metal pins to touch the client's scalp or face as they become hot under the dryer and can burn.

Rollers can also be placed off their base if a softer, flatter effect is required.

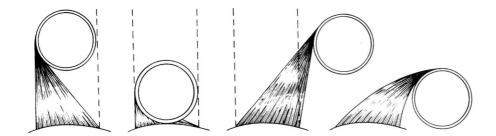

Rollers set on/off their base

Practise rollering with short, medium and long hair and placing rollers both on and off base for different effects.

Setting with pin curls

Pin curls are used to produce height, wave movement and curl in the finished dressing. They are usually secured with double-pronged clips, but care must be taken when securing them so that they do not become distorted.

Pin curls are made by turning around the ends of small, square sections of hair using the fingers to form a curl.

If one row of pin curls is placed in one direction (anti-clockwise curl) and the next row is placed in the opposite direction (clockwise curl), it is called reverse pin curling.

REMEMBER

The roller size chosen for each pli (set) will vary according to:
● the style chosen
● the amount of curl already in the hair
● the length and amount of hair
● the elasticity of the hair (some hair has very little elasticity and needs smaller rollers than usual).

REMEMBER

Rollers placed on their base give root lift. Rollers placed off their base give no root lift.

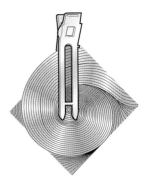

The most common type of pin curl: a **barrelspring curl**

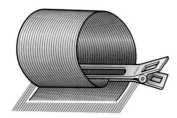

*Stand-up **barrel curl***

When you are working at the back and sides of the head, always ask your client to move their head forwards or to the side when necessary so that you can work properly.

Stand-up barrel curls

These are formed to give the same effect as you would achieve from using a roller, often where the space between the rollers is too small for another roller to fit.

Flat barrelspring curls

These pin curls are placed flat to the head to produce soft curls.

If one row of pin curls is placed in one direction and the next row is placed in the opposite direction, it is called reverse pin curling. These curls will brush out to form a wave movement.

TO DO

Practise each type of pin curl on short and medium hair.

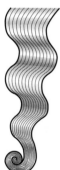

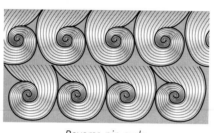

Reverse pin curls

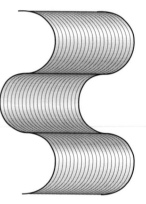

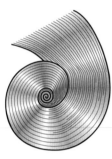

Clockspring curls

Clockspring curls

These are small, flat pin curls with a closed centre. The ends of the curl form a small closed circle with each loop becoming larger. They are normally used in the nape to produce tight curls.

Long-stemmed pin curls

These are useful for creating soft curl results around the hairline. As only the ends of the hair are curled, they are often secured to the skin with special sticky tape.

Finger waving

Finger waving is a way of moulding the hair with your fingers and salon comb to form a series of 'S'-shaped movements in the hair. It is best done on wet hair, but is also used on dry hair during combing out.

Points to remember for finger waving

Finger waving is best done on medium length, tapered hair that is not too curly.

- Keep the hair very wet. Use a thick setting gel to help form the waves.
- Always find the client's natural fall or parting and any natural wave movement, and finger wave with this movement. The hair should just fall into place.
- Use the wide teeth of the salon comb to comb the hair as these teeth penetrate the hair better.

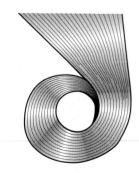

Long-stemmed pin curl

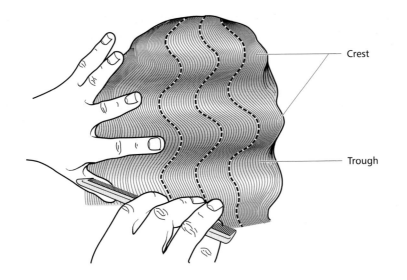

Crest

Trough

Finger waving

To form the 'S'-shaped movements start by combing the hair into a semi-circular shape, to form the trough of the wave. Then hold the hair in the centre of the wave in place with the middle and index fingers, while you comb the next section of hair into a semi-circular shape (in the opposite direction) to form the **crest** of the wave.

> **TO DO**
> *Practise finger waving on any clients who can spare the time before setting their hair.*

Variations of sets

There are many different ways of placing both rollers and pin curls to create different effects.

There are two methods of winding the hair.

Croquinole winding

Croquinole winding is used when volume, lift and movement is required. The hair is wound from points to roots. This method is suited for short to medium hair lengths.

Spiral winding

Spiral winding gives volume with even curl movement from roots to ends. Suitable for medium to longer length hair. Hair is wound from roots to points to give **spiral curls**.

If you have long hair and wish to achieve a tight curl at the roots as well as the ends, then you can use Molten Browners and spirally wind the hair. For best results, use end papers on towel-dried hair and secure the root end by bending the curler over.

> **TO DO**
> *Practise spiral winding on long hair.*

Points

Croquinole winding

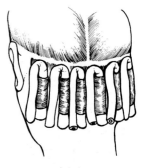

Spiral wind in position

Drying times

The approximate drying time depends upon the length of hair:

- short hair – approximately 10 minutes
- medium hair – approximately 10–20 minutes
- long hair – approximately 20–30 minutes.

Dry setting

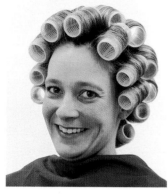

Dry setting

Fashion setting may be achieved on wet, damp or dry hair. The wetter the hair, the firmer and more long-lasting the set. Hair that is very wet and long takes a long time to dry, so more casual looks can be achieved on clean, dry hair. A thermal (heat active) styling lotion is then applied evenly and the hair may be set with either:

- heated rollers
- steam rollers or
- velcro rollers.

When using heated or steam rollers slightly larger sections are taken than for non-heated rollers.

Heated rollers retain their heat for approximately 10 to 15 minutes, and when they are completely cool, they should be removed from the client's hair.

Heated rollers

Heated rollers are used in much the same way as normal setting rollers. Available in a numbered set of specially designed wax fitted rollers in their own self-heating case, heated rollers use dry heat to soften and remould hair shapes. They are good for giving body and movement to straight and wavy hair. However, because these rollers contain heating elements and are pre-heated for several minutes prior to use, the hair must be completely dry. You must also ensure that none of the rollers come into contact with the client's skin by placing a piece of cotton wool on the area, i.e. ears and neck, before the roller is placed to ensure client safety.

Steam rollers

Steam rollers are also to be used on dry hair. The pre-heated steam rollers have a vented core that is wrapped with sponge. This allows steam to penetrate, to break the water bonds and remould the hair shape. Steam rollers gives stronger set shapes and prevent dehydration. They are suitable for fine, resistant hair, but are not recommended for hair that reacts poorly to moisture, as this will reactivate the curl.

Velcro rollers

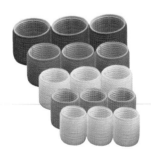

Velcro rollers

Velcro rollers gives soft wave curl movement. They are available in a variety of sizes and do not need pins. Velcro rollers are prone to tangling in longer hair lengths, so long hair needs to be held in place with clips. Hair coated in silicone styling products can reduce tangling.

The client's hair must be thoroughly dry. Spray each section of hair with the appropriate lotion before the roller is put into the hair.

After the hair has been completely set with rollers, place the client under a warm, pre-heated dryer (for 10–15 minutes).

Setting tight, curly hair

Naturally tight, curly hair is normally set after either temporary straightening (soft or hard pressing) or permanent straightening (relaxing) to create a modern fashion look. Hair that has been permed to create a tight, curly look may also be set when it is wet in order to create a softer style.

Patterns for setting

Here are some examples of different pli patterns. Notice that all the rollers are placed into a brickwork pattern – rollering in lines will only produce gaps and breaks in the comb out.

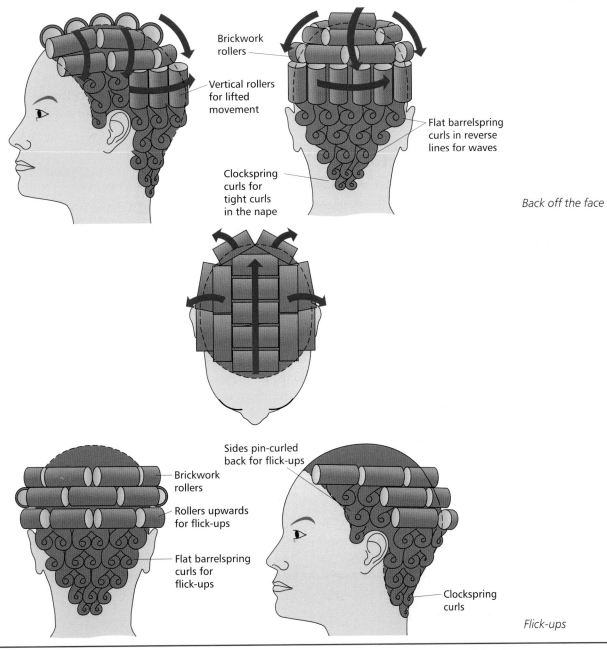

Brickwork rollers

Vertical rollers for lifted movement

Clockspring curls for tight curls in the nape

Brickwork rollers

Flat barrelspring curls in reverse lines for waves

Back off the face

Sides pin-curled back for flick-ups

Brickwork rollers

Rollers upwards for flick-ups

Flat barrelspring curls for flick-ups

Clockspring curls

Flick-ups

Hair can be set in order to:

- increase volume or
- decrease volume.

Increased hair volume can be achieved by:

- using large rollers, accompanied by a firm setting lotion or mousse with the addition of an amount of backcombing during dressing out of the set. This method is useful for adding height to the top of the head
- using small sections, small rollers and strong setting products, using some '**teasing**' in the dressing out of the hair to create voluminous curled effects.

Decreased hair volume can be achieved by:

- placing large rollers into the hair 'off base' with a 'drag' at the root area and not using any setting products that would give unwanted volume.

Combing out (dressing the hair)

Wella

Check that the hair is dry, then allow the hair to cool for a few minutes before removing the rollers. Always take the rollers out from the underneath first if the hair is long or it may become tangled.

Important factors

- Care must be taken not to scratch the client's scalp, ears or face.
- Be aware of the client's jewellery, i.e. earrings, getting caught in the brush or comb.
- Loosen the pli to remove any roller marks by brushing it out using a wide-bristle brush, e.g. vent or Denman brush, in all directions, then brush in the direction of the style before combing and teasing commences, particularly in the case of very small rollers/strong setting products.
- Always start brushing out at the nape area, gradually working up and around the head and finally brushing the hair off the face.
- Arrange the hair into the desired shape with the brush, before dressing it out with the comb. Only back-comb or back-brush where necessary.
- Some clients prefer a perfectly finished dressing, while others like a more casual result. The final dressing is what the client is paying for, so make sure that they are satisfied with the result.

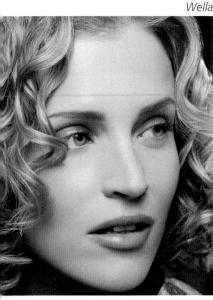

Dressing the hair

TO DO

- Re-read the section on pages 130–131 on finishing products. Hair sprays, gels, waxes, pomades, dressing creams, moisturisers, serums and activators may also be used before and after dressing out hair.
- Check all your manufacturers' instructions regarding the use of finishing products – many have to be used sparingly.

Back-brushing and back-combing

Both of these techniques work by pushing the cuticle scales apart so they tangle with each other. Both methods give lift and volume to the hairstyle.

Hold the points or ends of the hair firmly in one hand and either back-comb underneath or back-brush on top. Then gently smooth over the top to give a neat finish.

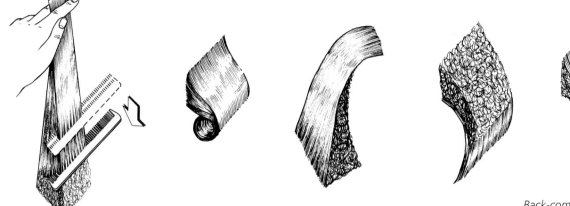

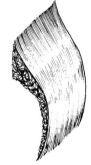

Back-combing technique

Always stand some distance away from your client to check the finished result, especially the shape. Look for any breaks or gaps in the dressing and smooth over if necessary.

Check the overall shape, looking at the back, sides and front. Does it frame the face properly? Remember that the client sees only the front area. It is the most important part of the dressing.

Hairspray and aerosol spray shines may now be used to finish the work and hold the shape.

TO DO

Practise showing clients the back of their hair using the back mirror. It should be held so that you can both see the back view.

Hairstyle maintenance assessment

Coarse/thick hair
- Ideal for styles with volume and movement.
- Requires softening and smoothing for straighter sleek styles.

Normal/medium hair
- Ideal for any style, straight or curly.
- Requires little or minimum work.

Fine/smooth hair
- Good for straight, sleek styles.
- Requires support and movement for voluminous styles.

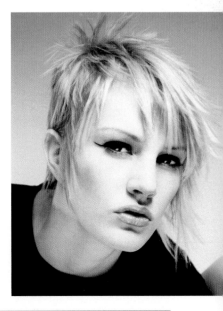

Dressing out long hair

Many hairdressers worry about working with long hair, but with planning and practice it does become easy.

TO DO

Using your style book and a long-haired practice head, follow the instructions in this book and practise plaiting, a pleat and a roll. Ask your supervisor to comment on your work.

Client consultation

- Use your style book to discuss the required style with your client and select the type of dressing most suitable.
- Discuss the occasion with your client. Is it for evening wear or for a wedding? Will you need extra-holding sprays for bad weather?
- Discuss the clothes your client will be wearing. Do they have a high or a low neckline? Will the hairstyle balance with the clothes?
- How much time will you need to dress the style? The client will not want to be late for a special occasion.
- Discuss the cost. Many salons charge extra for putting long hair up.
- For a very special occasion such as a wedding, have a rehearsal dressing beforehand to make sure you know exactly what the client wants.

General points

You will need to consider the following:

- the shape of the head – e.g. if it is flat at the back more hair will be needed there to balance it
- the shape of the face – e.g. if a round or square face is exposed by the hair being dressed up, then a few tendrils of hair around the face may be used to soften it
- the hair density (i.e. the amount of hair) and the length of the hair – does the client have enough hair for the dressing or will a hairpiece be needed?
- hair growth patterns – e.g. a widow's peak could be exposed if the client's hair is pulled back, so it may be softer to take the hair to the side
- hair texture – fine, frizzy hair may need wax, moisturisers or dressing cream to smooth it. Strong, coarse hair may need a strong styling lotion for control
- hair structure – e.g. if the hair is very straight will it need to be set first? If the hair is very curly will it need to be straightened first?

Preparation

Gowning up
Remove any large earrings or necklaces that the client is wearing, in case they become entangled in the client's long hair.

Freshly washed hair is difficult to dress so use a styling lotion during drying for control.

During dressing, products such as dressing creams (to remove frizz), wax and gels (to define the shape) and finishing spray (to hold the hair) are invaluable – but use them sparingly.

Equipment

Covered elastics and grips with covered ends are used to prevent hair damage, and should be kept to a minimum. This is because they should not show in the finished dressing and too many grips would be too heavy to wear comfortably.

Ornamentation

If you are using ornaments, such as combs, slides, flowers, ribbons or head-dresses in your dressing choose them carefully and make sure they balance the style rather than overwhelm it.

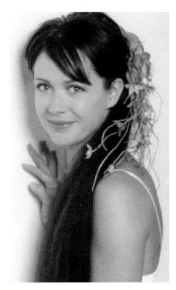

Ornamentation

Dressing hair down

- To dress out straight hair, simply brush it in place using your hands to create a smooth finish.
- To dress out curly hair, use your fingers or an afro comb to shape the hair. If you use a brush it will become frizzy.

Dressing hair up

Plaiting

Plaiting is a method of intertwining pieces of hair on the head with hair growing from the scalp or from added hair.

The two basic plaiting effects are plaits that hang from the head (free flowing) or those that cling to the scalp.

- A scalp plait uses thick stems taken from the head, with no parting.
- Corn row plaits use many parallel partings, with fine stems. Both these types of plaits create plaits that cling to the scalp.
- Added hair plaited to hair growing from the scalp can make hair appear longer, thicker and different.
- Free-flowing plaits are produced on the hair length. Thick stems, divided from the head with no parting, create a single, free-flowing plait. Thin stems, with many small partings over the scalp, create numerous free-flowing plaits over the head.
- Stem sizes and variety of the sections can influence the finished plait result.

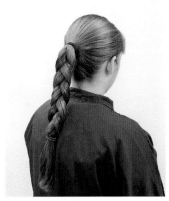

Single loose plait

Advice on plaiting

The hair is normally blow dried first using a styling product for control. Never over-dry the hair – it will lose its natural moisture content.

- Styling gels can be applied before plaiting to help retain neatness.
- Shine sprays applied to plaited hair help soften and moisturise the hair and scalp as well as shine.
- Layers in the hair can make plaiting difficult to achieve unless 'over-plaiting' is used. This method takes the 'ends' of the layers into the plait formation.
- If the hair is to be twisted or plaited, it must be brushed or combed smoothly and then divided into equal amounts.

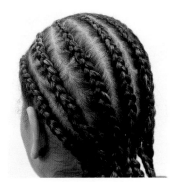

Corn row plaits

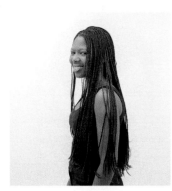

Many single, loose plaits

- Plaits can be achieved with more than three stems. An increased number of stems can produce beautiful results. Styles using six stems or more are referred to as woven hairstyles. The hairstyle resembles a basket weave.

- Hair twisted into tiny **braids** can, after the initial plaiting process, be left on the head for more than two months before they need to be removed.

- Plaited ends should be secured with covered bands, which can be elasticated.

- Uncoated rubber bands are not suitable, as these can split and tear the hair cuticle, and this can cause hair damage.

- Plaits are removed by unsecuring the ends and unravelling the plait from the end points to the root. This can be a time-consuming task, depending upon the number of plaits attached to the head.

TO DO

Use the illustrations below to practise making twists and plaits.

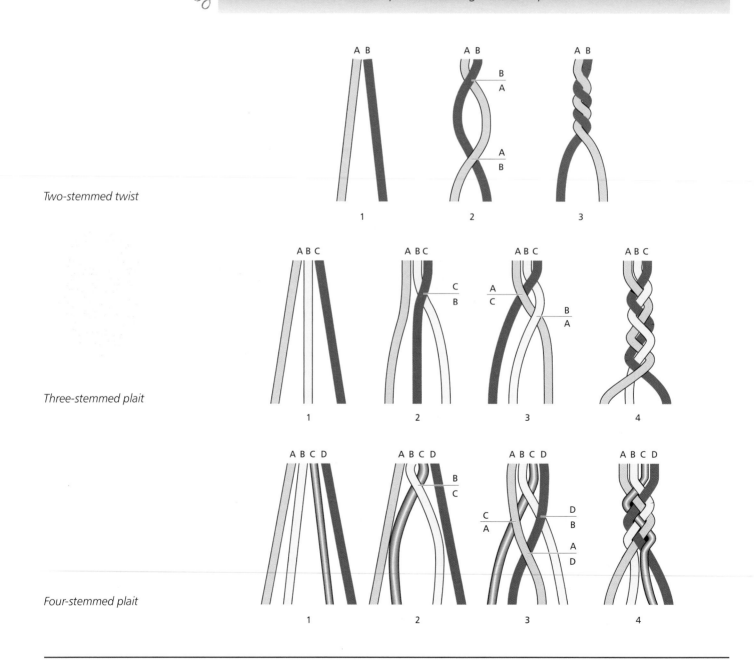

Two-stemmed twist

Three-stemmed plait

Four-stemmed plait

BASIC HAIRDRESSING

French (scalp) plait

A French plait is a three-stemmed plait, best done on dry hair. Starting at the front hairline, take a small triangular section and split the hair into three equal sections.

Work up to Diagram 3 of the three-stemmed plait diagram, then take another small section of hair from the right-hand hairline and add it to B/A. Pull the plait tight to the scalp. Next, take another small section from the left-hand hairline, keeping the hair combed smooth to the head, and add it to C/B. Pull the hair tight to the scalp. Continue adding small sections of hair to the plait until the French plait is completed.

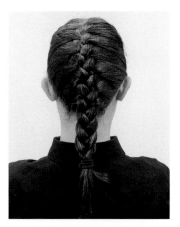

French plait

Pleats

A **pleat** is a vertical roll of hair worn at the back of the hair.

You should wet, dry or damp set the hair first on medium or large rollers to give some lift. The wetter the hair the more curly it will be.

Method

Back-comb or back-brush to create volume, control and to hold the hair together. Back-comb underneath the hair section at the roots and a little at the mid length and ends (Figure 1).

Leave out the top section and brush or comb (using the wide teeth) one side of the hair smoothly towards the centre back. Secure with a line of interlocking grips, placing one grip over the end of the last, firmly to the scalp. Finish the line of grips just under the crown area. If you are right-handed, it is easier to secure the left side first (Figure 2).

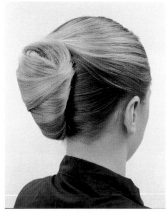

A pleat

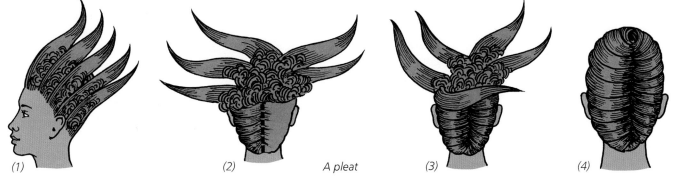

(1) (2) *A pleat* (3) (4)

Brush or comb the other side of the hair across towards the centre back. Check that the pleat is in the middle, then twist or fold this hair under and secure firmly with grips or pins, making sure that they do not show (Figure 3).

Smooth over the top hair and blend it in with the pleated back hair, completing the pleat smoothly and tucking in the ends (Figure 4). Grip it firmly, then check the front of the dressing for balance and shape. If the hair needs lifting use a pin or the end of a tail comb carefully so as not to disturb the hair that is already secured. Use finishing spray as desired. Check that no pins or grips are visible.

Traction alopecia

Traction alopecia is caused when excessive tension is applied to the hair. It generally occurs in women who wear severe hairstyles and happens only when the traction is prolonged; in which case the hair is pulled out at the roots, especially along the front hairline, sides and partings.

When the cause of the tension is removed, the hair usually grows back, although, if traction has been applied over a long period of time, then the hair loss may be permanent.

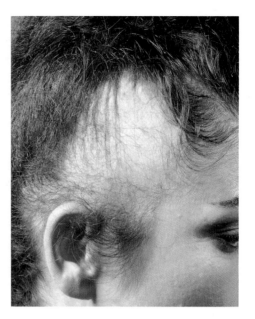

Traction alopecia

The area around the front hairline is an important factor to consider before commencing a plait. If it is fine or sparse, it may be difficult to produce a good plait.

Added hair (postiche)

This is when either real or synthetic hairpieces are added into the hairstyle and may cover all or part of the head. Add-ons include clip-on pony-tails and fringes. Other types of added hair (**postiche**) are extensions and weaves. Full wigs pull over the scalp to cover all the client's own hair.

Add-ons

Add-ons such as ponytails and wiglets can be used to hide sparse areas, or add volume and lift. Natural hair and add-on hair should be intertwined together to hide the joins and they must be securely clipped or combed into the hair.

Extensions and weaves

Extensions and weaves are not just for those losing their hair or for hiding sparse areas.

Extensions involve plaiting, knotting (usually synthetic hair) or melting specialised bonds (human hair) in tiny amounts to similar amounts of the natural hair. They can be longer for length or shorter for volume and lift.

Weaves are more complicated; these are sewn on to the hair. The natural hair is scalp plaited into pattered corn rows that form the foundation or base of the weave. The weave wefts are then sewn on to the corn rows.

As with extensions, the process is time consuming and maintenance is regularly required as the weave loosens when the natural hair grows, and it needs to be re-tightened.

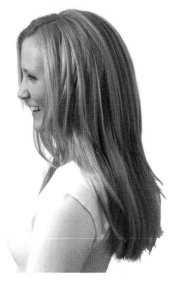

Synthetic hair

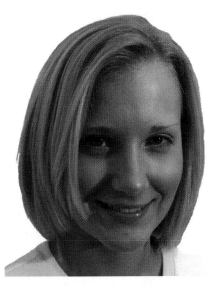

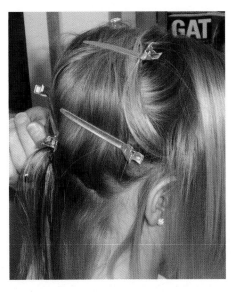

Process of weaves

Weaves are ideal when clients want their hair to take a rest from chemical treatments and constant physical blow drying or straightening.

They are also ideal for a short-to-long hair length change without the cutting of natural hair.

Note that clients with fine hair who require added hair need special attention to check whether their hair is strong enough to support the extra weight.

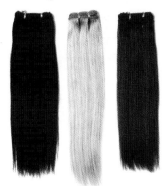

Human hair

Wigs

- Wigs should closely match own hair colour for a natural look.
- Real hair is more expensive, but can be processed, although it is important to find out what was already done to the hair, so as not to weaken it.
- Synthetic hair is easy to clean, hardwearing and inexpensive compared to real hair, although it cannot be processed and it can look false.
- Advise clients not to keep the wig on the head longer than needed, but always allow their own hair and scalp to breathe, as the wig will trap moisture and heat. It should also be remembered that the tension stress that wigs put on the hair can cause traction alopecia.
- The placing of the wig is all-important and, most importantly, it should be wrapped with natural hair from the hairline to help conceal and match the style.

FAULT	CAUSE	CORRECTION
'Fishhooks' or **buckled,** frizzy ends	Ends of hair not wound smoothly around the rollers	Try using electric tongs to smooth out the hair. 'Fishhooks' will disappear as soon as the hair is wetted down
Hair not dry	Incorrect checking	Replace rollers and re-dry the hair under the dryer. If brushed through, then dry with a hand-held dryer and small circular brush
Hair not curly enough	Rollers too large	Use electric tongs to tighten the curl
Hair too curly	Rollers too small	Use hand dryer and brush to stretch the hair straighter
Hair is greasy and lank	Conditioner left in the hair or too much spray shine applied	The hair must be re-shampooed and set again
Hair is flyaway and full of static electricity	Too much shampoo used, or the hair is naturally flyaway	Apply a little spray shine to the hair. Use a setting aid next time
Holes and breaks in the hair in final comb out	Too few rollers. Not enough brushing or combing out	Re back-comb or back-brush the area of hair

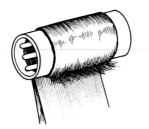

Overlapping ends

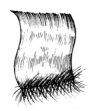

'Fishhooks'

TEST YOUR KNOWLEDGE

1 What effect does the size of rollers have on the finished style?
2 What are the benefits of using too many rather than too few rollers when setting?
3 What are the effects of using:
   - small rollers
   - large rollers
   - small rollers and clockspring pin curls
   - large rollers on top and smaller rollers underneath?
4 Why is the natural fall and root movement so important when designing the pli?
5 What happens to the temporary bonds in the cortex during cohesive (wet) setting?
6 Why does a set collapse on a damp, misty day?
7 List and compare different types of styling and drying equipment for use on tight curly, wavy and straight hair.
8 Describe which of the following products:
   - setting lotion
   - sculpting or moulding mists or lotions
   - mousse
   - gel

   would be suitable for setting (a) fine hair, (b) coarse hair, (c) tight curly hair, (d) wavy hair, (e) straight hair, (f) soft sets, (g) tight sets.
9 Why should set hair sections be brushed out thoroughly before dressing and styling the hair?
10 List and compare different types of equipment and finishing products for use on tight curly, wavy and straight hair to achieve various looks.
11 Describe the type of products, equipment and ornamentation used for dressing tight curly, wavy and straight long hair into different styles.
12 Why should clients who have their hair regularly plaited be warned about traction alopecia?
13 Describe the four main types of added hair (postiche).

Chapter 7 Cutting

After working through this chapter you will be able to:

- Maintain effective and safe methods of working
- Cut hair into shape using three basic techniques
- Understand how hair growth patterns, density and hair type can affect the tools and techniques used
- Understand the different cutting techniques and when to use them
- Know the tools available for use and how to use them.

This chapter covers the following NVQ Level 2 unit:
Cut Hair Using Basic Techniques

More clients visit the hairdresser for cutting than for any other service, because it is impossible for an untrained person to achieve as good a cut. A good haircut is the basis of every hairstyle and can completely change clients' views of themselves.

The hairdresser can remove both length and thickness by cutting, and create a completely new shape or style.

Gowning up

TO DO

Check with your supervisor to see if your salon has any particular requirements for gowning up for a:
- *wet cut*
- *dry cut*
- *man's cut*
- *woman's cut*
- *child's cut.*

There is nothing more irritating for a client than leaving the salon covered in pieces of hair. Hairs not only fall down the back of clothing but get stuck in all sorts of fabrics and clothes (especially sweaters) and are difficult to remove. So it is important to gown up properly.

Gowns are used to cover the client's clothes, and shoulder capes can be used around the client's shoulders. Clean towels may be placed around the client's neck during wet cutting, but, as cut hairs embed themselves into towels, it is more hygienic to towel dry the hair and use cutting collars for protection.

To prevent cut hairs from falling into the client's clothing, insert a strip of cotton wool or neck tissue around the neck area. These are disposable and should be used only once.

Wet-cut hairs are especially difficult to remove from the skin, but the use of talcum powder and a neck brush makes their removal easier.

Always keep a clothes brush at reception to remove hairs from the client's clothes after the gown and cape are removed, and remember to clean your work area by brushing loose, cut hairs into the waste area as soon as you are finished.

TO DO

- Re-read the section in Chapter 3 on the disposal of waste materials – ask your supervisor if the procedure for your salon is the same.
- Re-read the section on designing a hairstyle to suit your client in Chapter 1.

Advantages of cutting hair dry

REMEMBER

Wet hair stretches much more than dry hair and when it dries it can become very much shorter.

- Hair is not as elastic or stretchy as when wet, so you can see its true length as you cut.
- You can see split ends clearly to cut them off (see Chapter 5).
- It is easier to use electric **clippers** on dry hair.
- The client may not have enough time or money for a wet cut, but may be willing to have a dry trim.
- If you are **thinning** the haircut with special **thinning scissors** you will remove less hair when it is dry.

Advantages of cutting hair wet

- The hair is clean and not as tangled as it is when dry (easier to comb).
- You can see the natural fall clearly only when the hair is wet.
- Precision cutting is always done on wet hair because cutting **guide lines** can be seen clearly.
- More varied cutting techniques, e.g. **razor cutting** and slide cutting, can be used on wet hair.

Hair thickness and waviness

Fine and coarse hair

See the section in Chapter 1 (page 11), which covers the different thicknesses of hair. Very thin or fine hair can be difficult to cut because, unless you are careful, 'steps' can appear.

On the other hand, some hair is so coarse and wiry that only very sharp tools (scissors and razors), used on fine sub-sections, will cut it easily.

Curly and straight hair

To remind you, there are three main racial hair types:

- European – generally wavy
- Asian (including Chinese and Japanese hair) – usually straight
- African Caribbean – very curly.

All types of hair need to be cut differently.

Generally, **straight** hair must be cut carefully or '**steps**' will appear, and more movement can be produced by layering and thinning.

People with **curly** hair will find that if their long hair is cut short it will appear even curlier! This is because the weight of long hair stretches it and it appears more wavy than curly.

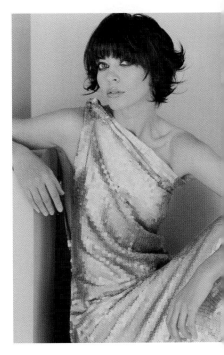

Weight distribution and the natural fall of hair

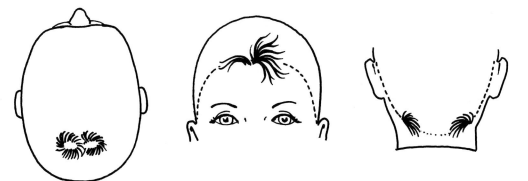

Double crown   *Cowlick*   *Neck whorl*

Distribution of hair lies naturally forward from the crown; frequent combing of the hair can train the hair to fall in different positions.

Strong hair growth patterns and natural falls are difficult to retrain. To ignore these natural growth patterns and falls will result in unattractive or unmanageable hairstyles.

TO DO

Re-read the section in Chapter 5 on hair growth patterns, noting how to cut hair with:

- a double crown
- a cowlick
- a nape whorl
- a widow's peak.

TEST YOUR KNOWLEDGE

1. State how the following critical factors can influence your choice of haircut:
   - hair structure
   - hair texture
   - head and face shape
   - hair growth patterns.

2. Give examples of how you would advise your client to select a suitable style.

3. Why is it important to keep your work area clean and tidy and avoid cross-infections and infestations?

Cutting tools

All cutting tools must be sharp, in good condition, clean and sterile, and should never be kept in pockets or left around out of their case.

These are the most commonly used tools in cutting.

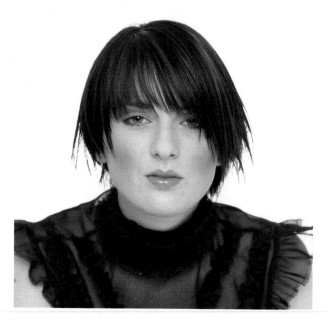

Wella

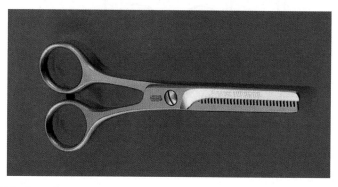

Thinning scissors

Scissors

Good-quality scissors are made of well-tempered or cobalt steel and are available in various sizes – from 10 cm to 18 cm from the tip of the blade to the handles. Many hairdressers prefer to use short scissors for precision cutting, but long scissors are useful for other techniques such as those used for cutting African Caribbean hair and barbering.

Looking after your scissors

- Never use them for cutting anything other than hair – they will quickly become blunt.
- After removing any cut hairs, always keep the blades dry by wiping them with cotton wool and surgical spirit (this will also disinfect the blades).

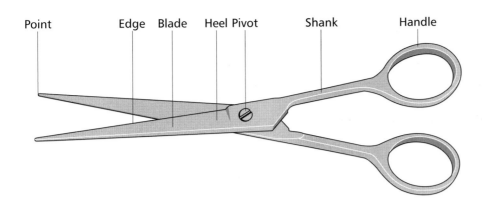

The parts of scissors

- Lightly oil the blades and the pivot screw if they start to feel stiff and awkward to use.
- Try not to drop your scissors – the blades may be damaged and the pivot screw (which balances the scissors) could work loose.
- Keep your scissors in their original protective case for safety and to prevent them being damaged.
- If your scissors need mending or sharpening, always send them to a professional hairdressing scissors company (advertisements are found in hairdressing trade journals).

REMEMBER

Scissors are very expensive. Look after them properly.

TO DO

- *Re-read the section in Chapter 3 (page 55) on the sterilisation of tools and equipment.*
- *List and describe the four different methods of sterilisation.*

HEALTH MATTERS

Choose your scissors carefully – they must fit the size of your hand and feel comfortable to work with. Try asking different stylists in your salon if you may hold their scissors to see how they feel.

During cutting keep your wrist in a straight line from middle finger to elbow, to prevent wrist strain. Before starting a haircut always adjust the height of your chair or bend from your knees, keeping your back straight to make sure you are not bending incorrectly. Face forwards and look down slightly. If your head is slanted too much it means that its weight is being supported by your neck muscles instead of your bones and this can result in strain, neck pain or headaches. A cutting stool is an excellent idea as it allows you to work at the correct height and can be moved from side to side around the client.

Holding your scissors

You can always spot a professional hairdresser by the way they pick up and hold a pair of scissors using their thumb and third finger. They do this to achieve maximum control during cutting.

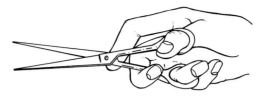

Holding the scissors

Scissor handling exercises

These exercises are necessary to help you become familiar with the weight and feel of the scissors. They will also help you to move the blades of the scissors into many positions.

- Holding the scissors inbetween the fingers, aim the points towards the opposite hand and place the bottom blade on the hand.
- Moving the top blade only, open and close the blades.

With practice this exercise should be conducted without resting the blade on the hand.

- Correctly holding the scissors inbetween the fingers, hold the arm upright, balancing the elbow on a flat surface.
- Using the wrist only, slowly move the scissor points left to right.
- Then open and close the blades while moving the scissors slowly from left to right using the wrist.

Combs

Cutting combs are normally used during cutting. One end of the comb has close-set teeth; one end has wider-set teeth. When cutting, the hair can be held firmly in place by this comb prior to cutting a straight line. They are also used to scissor over comb cutting. A fine, flexible barber's comb can be used if you need to cut really short neck hairs.

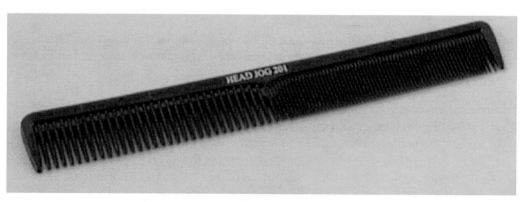

Cutting comb

During cutting, the sub-section of hair to be cut is held in the fingers of one hand and the scissors in the other. To hold the comb at the same time, palm the scissors for safety and hold the comb in your scissor hand.

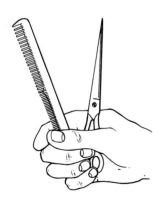

Palming the scissors

TO DO

Practise taking your thumb out of the scissor handles, closing the scissors and holding the comb at the same time.

BASIC HAIRDRESSING

Cutting techniques using scissors

Club cutting

Club cutting this is the most common cutting technique. However, it must be precise and for this reason is often called precision cutting.

The sub-section of hair must be cleanly combed through and held with an even tension before cutting.

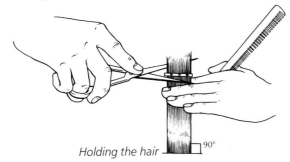

Holding the hair — 90°

The diagram shows hair cut at 90° for a layer cut, but the hair may be cut at any angle to the head according to the style planned. Club cutting may be done on wet or dry hair and the ends of the hair are left blunt and heavy (this is sometimes also called **blunt cutting**).

Freehand cutting

This is where the hair is cut without being held in place with tension from any forced directional pull. The hair is combed from its section and allowed to fall into its own natural movement before cutting.

- It is a particularly useful technique during one-length cutting, where a straight line is required. On below shoulder-length hair, holding the hair with a finger underneath can cause unwanted **graduation**.
- Cutting fringes with a cowlick will naturally make the hair bounce up too short if it is cut with tension.

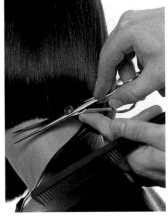

Freehand cutting

Taper cutting

Taper or slither cutting (**feathering**) will reduce both the length and the thickness of the hair. This technique is done on dry hair and, unlike club cutting (where the hair is cut over the fingers), the hair is cut underneath the fingers.

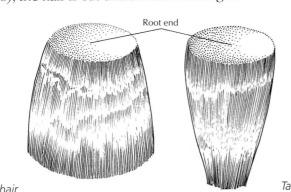

Root end

Club cut hair   *Taper cut hair*

Tapering is a sliding, slithering, backwards-and-forwards movement along a sub-section of hair. Close the scissor blades as you move towards the roots.

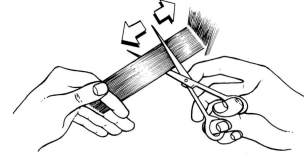

Tapering motion

TO DO

Practise the action of taper cutting by opening and closing your scissors in slow motion, at the same time moving the points of the scissors away from you, then back towards you.

Pointing and texturising

Pointing can be used to achieve feathered effects and to soften hard lines created by club cutting.

Take a sub-section of hair and insert the scissors over the fingers to chip out small pieces at the ends of the hair.

When larger pieces are taken out of the hair this is called texturising.

Scissor over comb

This technique is used to give the same effect as clipper over comb work – the hair around the nape and sides is cut short, following the contours of the head.

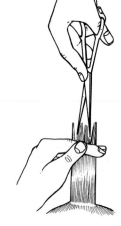

Pointing

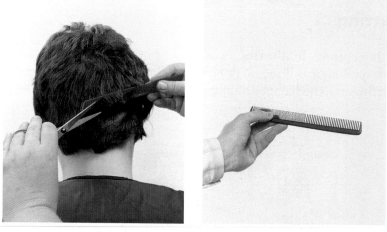

Scissor over comb

Holding the comb

Use a cutting comb to pick up the hair, keeping the scissors parallel to the comb during cutting. Use the comb in an upwards direction, lifting the hair sticking through it can be cut off. Move the comb and scissors continually towards the top of the head, keeping the comb up and out and away from the head, cutting at the same time.

Thinning hair with thinning scissors

These scissors remove only thickness or bulk from the hair, not length. They are sometimes called **aesculaps**, serrated or texturising scissors.

Ordinary thinning scissors can be used to thin out from the middle of the hair, cutting diagonally across the sub-section of the hair. Open and close them two or three times to remove the thickness.

Many new variations on the normal thinning scissors, with different shapes of blades to create lots of exciting effects, have been developed.

Cutting techniques using clippers and razors

Clippers

Electric clippers are now commonly used for both men's and women's hairdressing to give the same effect as the 'scissor over comb' technique. They have two blades with sharp-edged teeth. One blade remains fixed while the other moves across it. The action of the motorised moving blade is similar to several pairs of scissors being used at the same time, and many hairdressers like the speed of cutting with clippers.

Detachable clipper heads are available so that the closeness of the cut can be altered. The larger the number, the longer the length; the smaller the number, the shorter the length.

Razors

Two main types of razor are in use:
- an open or cut-throat razor
- a modern hair shaper or safety razor.

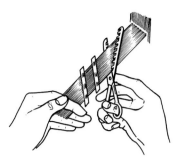

Thinning the hair with thinning scissors

REMEMBER

Use thinning scissors only on dry hair – you could thin the hair too much if the hair is wet.
Do not thin:
- around the hairline
- at the crown area
- too close to the scalp
- along any partings because spiky ends will result.

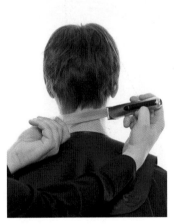

Clipper over comb technique

REMEMBER

Health and safety
The bottom, static blade of the clippers should always be further forward than the top, moving blade. If the top blade comes too far forwards you could cut someone's skin, so be extra careful when clippers are turned over for lining out. Always put on the blade guard when clippers are not in use.

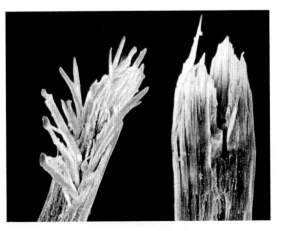

A hair that has been cut with a blunt razor

Both are used on wet hair because razoring on dry hair is painful for the client. Razors must be kept sharp or they will tear the hair.

REMEMBER

Keep clipper blades well oiled and free of cut hairs; clean them regularly.

Open or cut-throat razors

Open razors may be used to shorten the hair and to remove thickness. They are used underneath or above the wet sub-sections of hair and are stroked towards the ends with a scooping movement that produces a tapered effect. Many hairdressers also use open razors to create a clean hairline around the haircut.

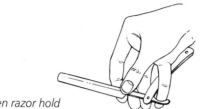
Open razor hold

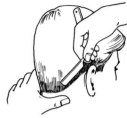
Hairline shaping

It is important to hold a razor safely so that it does not close up on your hand during cutting.

Open razors are now available with disposable blades. These are more hygienic, and as one blade becomes blunt you can replace it so you always have a sharp edge to use. Used disposable blades must be disposed of safely so that anyone handling waste does not cut themselves.

Shapers or safety razors

These razors have a guard over the blade so that only part of the hair is cut. They produce a feathered, uneven effect and are easier and safer to use than an open razor.

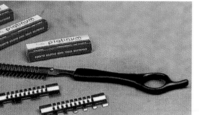
Safety razor

TO DO

The Health and Safety at Work Act 1974 requires you to work safely. Find the address of your local Health and Safety Executive (HSE) from your library or town hall and check the local by-laws regarding the use of razors, and the disposal of sharps (i.e used disposable razor blades).

Cutting tools and techniques

TECHNIQUE	TOOLS	CUT WET OR DRY	EFFECTS
Club cutting	Scissors Clippers	Wet or dry Dry	Removes length. Hair curls less. Ends of hair look thicker
Freehand cutting	Scissors	Wet or dry	Removes length or thickness within the natural fall of the hair
Taper cutting	Scissors Razor	Dry Wet	Removes length. Removes thickness. Hair curls more
Pointing and texturising	Scissors	Wet or dry	Removes thickness from the ends of the hair and can create a spiky, textured effect. Use to remove 'steps' in haircut
Scissor/clipper	Scissors	Dry	Removes length
Over comb	Clippers	Dry	Used for short, often graduated haircuts
Thinning	Thinning scissors Razor	Dry Wet	Removes thickness from the hair

Points to remember during cutting

- You must have checked in your mind that the style will suit the client, but also make sure that you and the client are talking about the same hairstyle. Use a photograph if necessary to double-check.
- Check the natural growths (crown area, natural partings, etc.) again. Try to work with the hair, not against it – the client has to manage the style at home without your help.
- Use section clips to keep large sections of hair apart so that you can work cleanly.

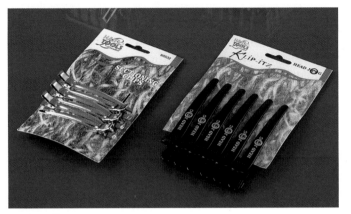

Section clip

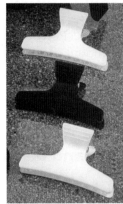

Butterfly clamp

- Keep your cutting sections small and narrow so that you can always see your guideline.
- Use an open-tufted brush (a vent brush) during cutting to brush the hair in different directions so you can see how well the hair is falling into shape.

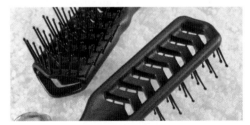

Vent brush

- Always keep a water spray close at hand to dampen the hair if it starts to dry.
- Use the mirrors around the salon to check the shape of the client's haircut from various angles.
- Hand mirrors can also be used to check short graduations or bobs by placing them directly underneath the hairline.
- Do not pull the hair or use too much tension around the ears or when cutting a fringe over a cowlick – it may bounce up too short. Use freehand cutting instead.
- Check your client's head position – is it level? If their legs are crossed, then their head will be lop-sided – and so will your haircut!
- To make sure that the sides are level take small strands of hair from either side and gradually slide your fingers to the ends. If the strands have been taken from exactly the same place at each side your thumbs will be level.
- Use parts of the face (nose and eyes) to check lengths are equal.
- Ask the client throughout the cutting, 'Is this the correct length?'

Cutting angles and lines for different styles

There are two types of cutting guide, as follows.

Stationary

The first cut is the cutting guide; all other hair sections are brought to this guideline and cut, e.g. one-length cut (see step 1 on page 170).

Travelling/moving

Each new section becomes the cutting guide; to ensure even layering and balance, a small amount of the first-cut hair mesh is held out with the second mesh and cut following the length of the first cut, e.g. uniform layered cuts (see step 5 on page 171).

Guidelines must be clearly seen when cutting; otherwise an uneven cut will result (see step 2 on page 170).

Angles and degrees of graduation

The two important **cutting angles** to take into account when cutting hair are:
- the angle at which the hair is held out from the head
- the angle at which the hair is cut (see step 4 on page 171).

These two angles decide the falling position of the hair on the head.

There are only three style plans, from which all other styles can be achieved:
- the one-length cut
- the layer cut
- the graduation (layers graduating from long to short).

The one-length cut

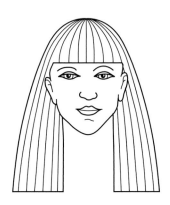

One-length cut

This is where the hair is cut to fall at the same outside length. Hair often looks thicker when cut in this style.

The guidelines are taken either horizontally or diagonally, starting at the hairline, and each section is taken parallel to the cutting line.

Always cut a one-length cut from the natural fall, from both the parting and the crown area, combing the hair perfectly smooth and even.

To check that a one-length cut is even, ask the client to slowly move their head from side to side and backwards and forwards. Any unevenness or long ends will be clearly visible.

A uniform layer cut

In a uniform layer cut all sections of the hair to the same length. The outline shape is cut first, and then the inner shape is cut by holding the hair up at 90°.

To check that the cut is even, comb the layers in the opposite direction to the way in which you have cut them. They must be perfectly even, with no long ends.

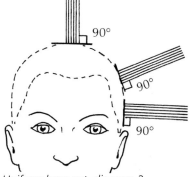

Uniform layer cut, diagram 1   Uniform layer cut, diagram 2

Graduated layers

Short graduated layers
In this cut, the inner layers of the hair lengths are longer than the outline shape (the outline hair length). It is cut using a combination of a one-length cut and scissor or clipper over comb cut.

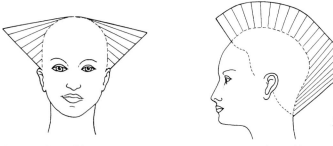

Short graduated layers   Long graduated layers

Long graduated layers
This is a long layer cut, sometimes known as reverse graduation, in which the inner layers of the hair lengths are shorter than the outline shape (the outline hair length).

The longer layers have to be over-directed (pulled upwards) to match the shorter layers, and then blended together.

 TO DO

Check with your supervisor and find out how long it should take you to cut:
- *a one-length cut*
- *a layer cut*
- *a short graduation*
- *a long graduation.*

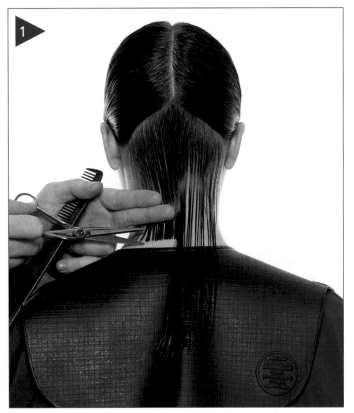

Back view stationary cutting guide

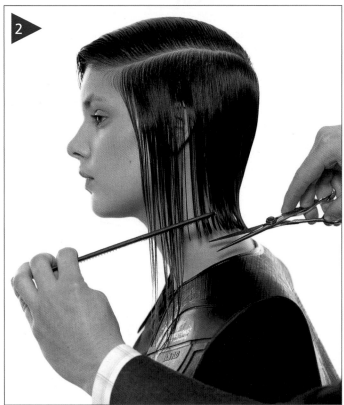

Side view, joining the back cutting guide to the side cutting guide

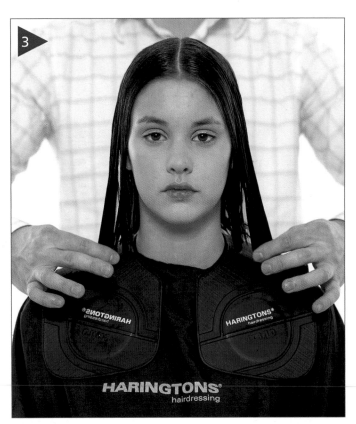

Balancing the haircut

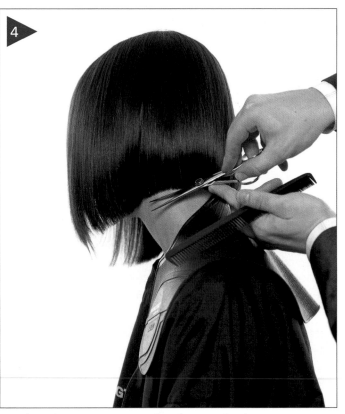

Freehand cutting against the skin on dry hair

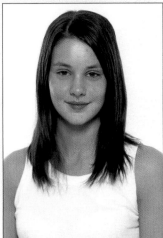

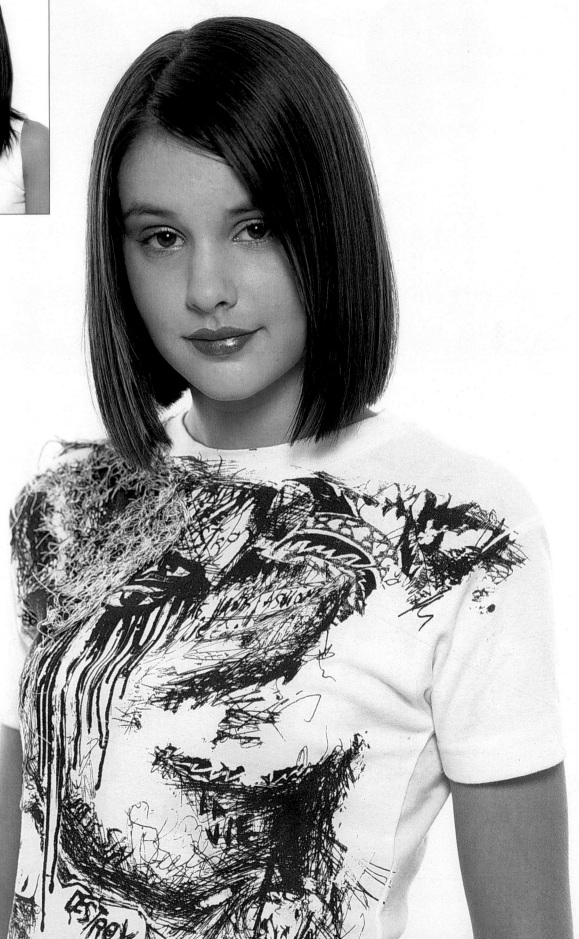

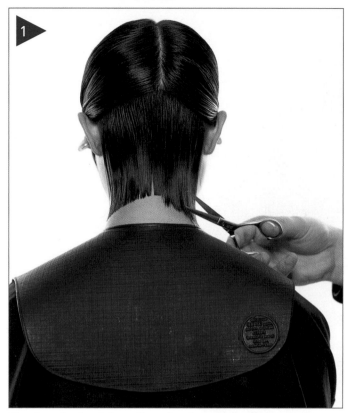

Cutting the back baseline, freehand

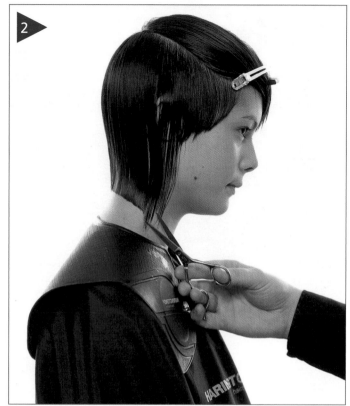

Cutting the side baseline, freehand

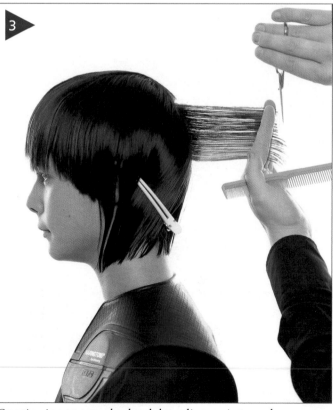

Continuing to use the back baseline as internal guideline, holding the hair at 90°

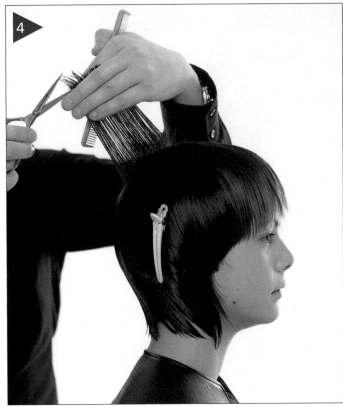

Using the internal guideline at the top of the head, holding the hair at 90° (side view)

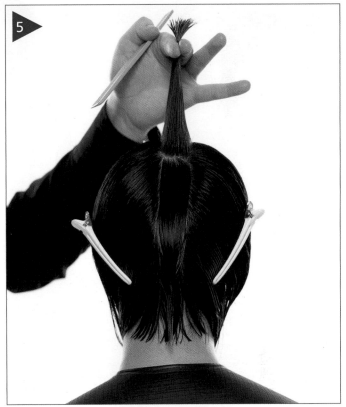

Using the internal guideline at the top of the head, holding the hair at 90° (back view)

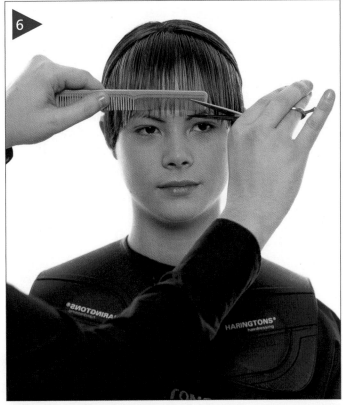

Cutting the front baseline fringe

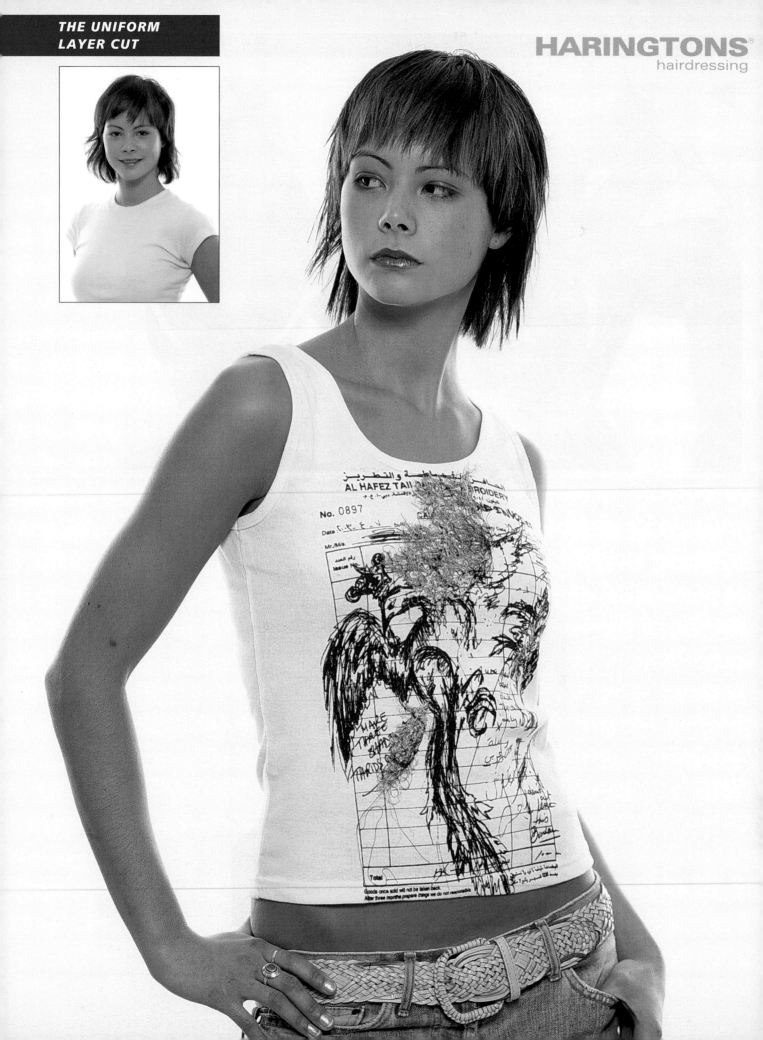

THE UNIFORM
LAYER CUT

HARINGTONS
hairdressing

HARINGTONS®
hairdressing

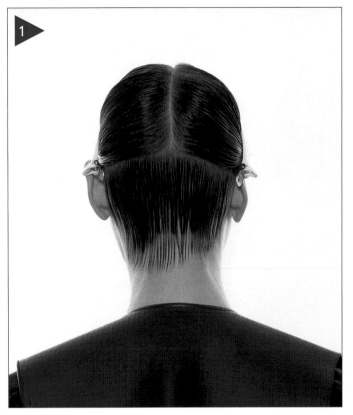

Hair sectioned above the occipital bone

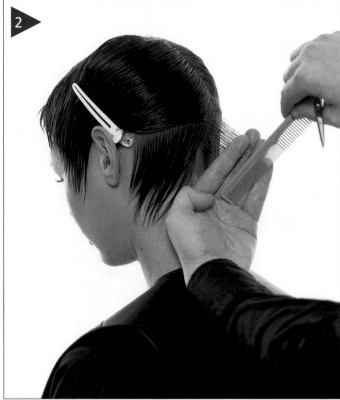

Graduating the first section underneath, holding the hair at 45°, using an internal guideline

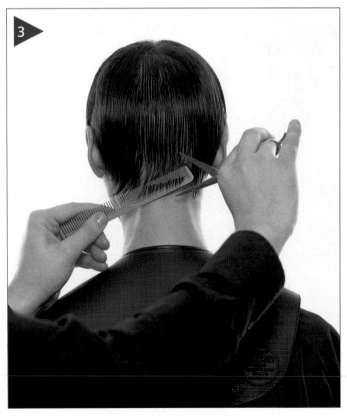

Scissor over combing the back baseline for a short graduation

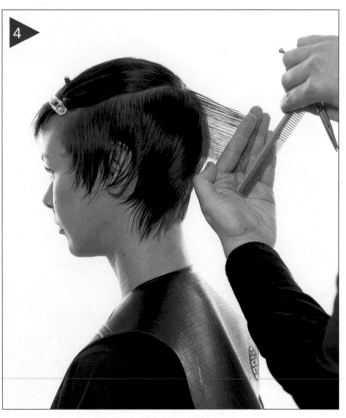

Continuing to graduate the back, holding hair at 45°, using an internal guideline

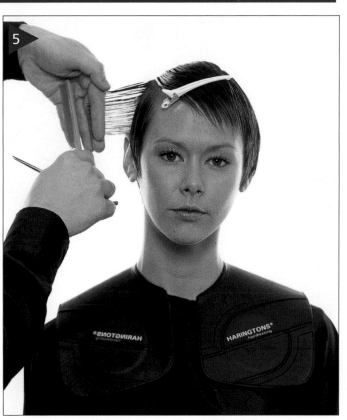

Continuing to graduate
the side of the hair at 45°

THE LONG GRADUATED LAYER CUT

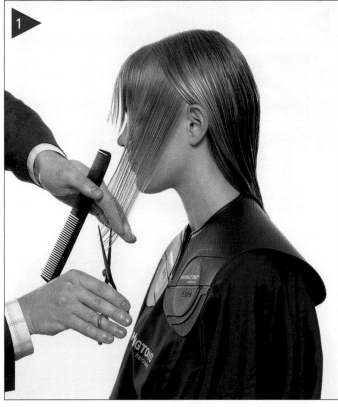

Cutting the side baseline by holding the hair down and
slightly forward

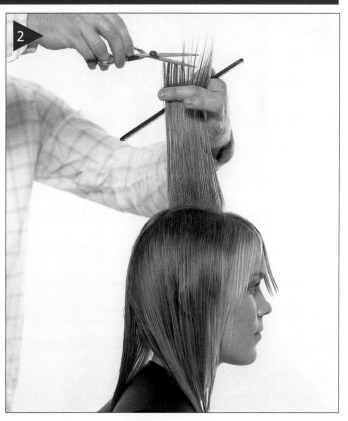

Creating the internal guideline for the long graduated
layers at the top of the head, holding the hair at 90°

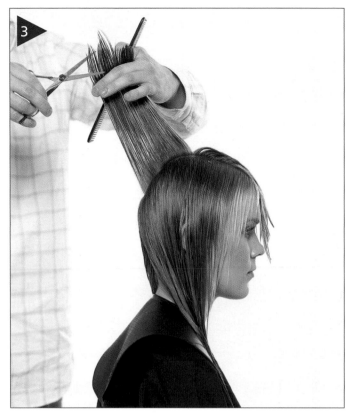

Joining the crown section to the internal guidelines, holding the hair at 90°

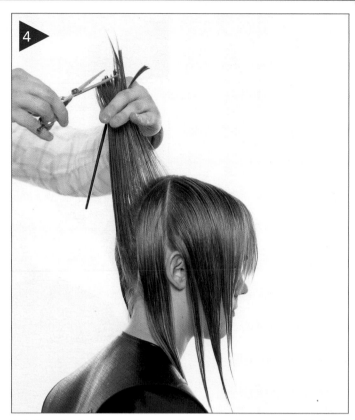

Joining the back section to the crown internal guideline by overdirecting the hair to create long graduated layers

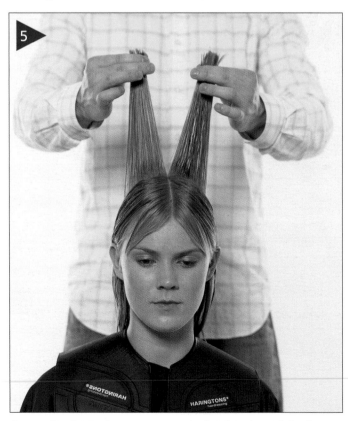

Cross checking the cut to ensure both sides of the long graduation are even

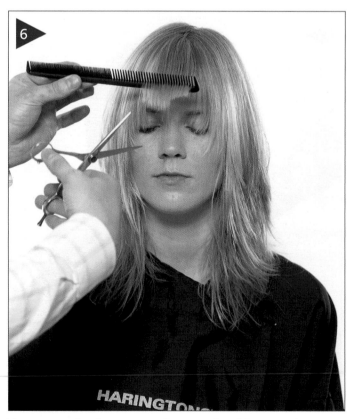

Texturising the fringe to soften any hard lines and create the finished look

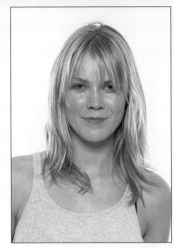

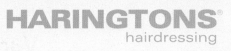

Variations in cuts

Front lines

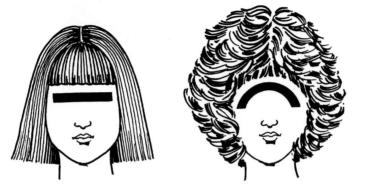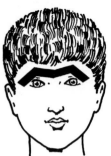

Side lines

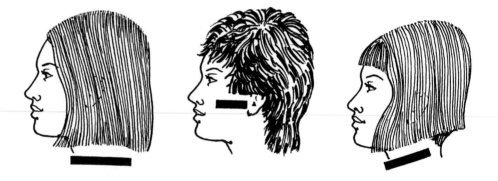

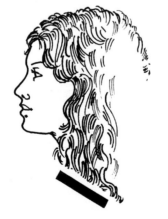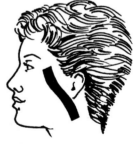

Back lines

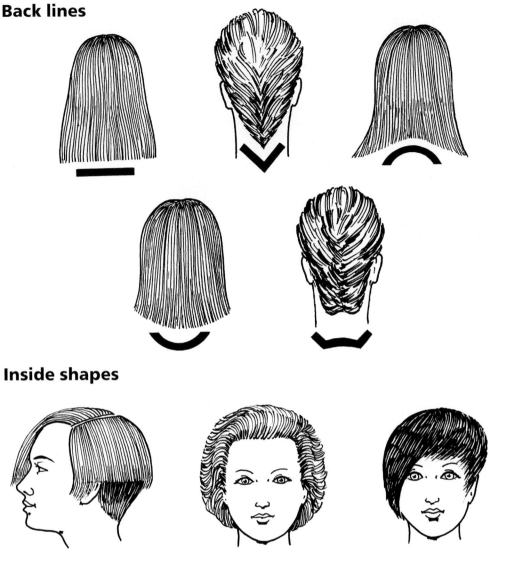

Inside shapes

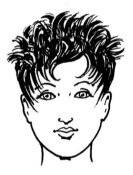

Achieving fashion looks

Once you have mastered the basic cutting methods and techniques you should be able to reproduce any of the latest fashion looks.

A guideline or a baseline is the cut section of hair that is used as a cutting guide for the next sections. You must always be able to see the guide – if you have lost it, it is because the next section was too thick, and you will need to re-section and start again from the guide.

Sometimes there is more than one guideline. For instance, with a short graduation, the one-length guideline is cut first – with the fingers resting on the head, the hair is cut to the same length all around the middle of the head. For the second guideline the underneath hair is cut at an angle from the nape and the sides, section by section, to meet the first guideline.

To combine cutting methods, the basic shape of the cut is produced first, often by club cutting, then other methods may be introduced on the same sections of hair to give different looks, e.g. a textured, tapered look.

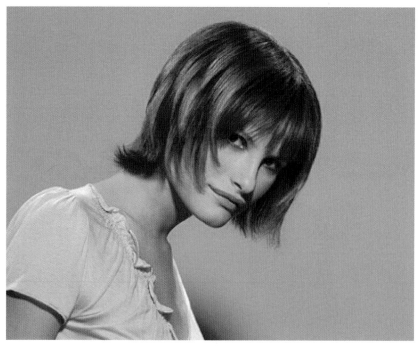

Textured bob

TO DO

- *Find four pictures of different current fashion looks for a friend, two one-length and two layered.*
- *Write up a description of how these were achieved, and why they would be suitable for your friend.*

Accidents when cutting

Accidentally cutting the client

REMEMBER

The skin on the ear lobes is quite thin, and a small cut may bleed more than expected, so ask the client to keep the pressure on until the blood clots.

If an accident does happen, keep calm and give the client a sterile dressing, asking them to apply this with pressure to the cut to stop bleeding. (Do not touch the cut yourself because of the health risks, such as HIV and hepatitis B.) Small cuts may be covered with a sterile dressing but larger cuts may need medical attention.

TO DO

Find out where the first aid box is in your salon and make sure there are plenty of sterile dressings and assorted plasters before you start cutting.

Accidentally cutting yourself

REMEMBER

Always record in the accident book any accidents that occur during cutting.

Many hairdressers cut themselves during haircutting (a common place is between the first and second fingers, where you hold the hair).

Stop whatever you are doing and excuse yourself from the client. Rinse the cut with water to remove any hairs, then apply pressure with a sterile dressing until the blood clots and the bleeding stops. Dry the area, then apply a sterile plaster.

BASIC HAIRDRESSING

After the haircut

Cross-checking

Cross-checking should be done after every haircut to make sure that it is level and evenly balanced from all angles.

Cross-checking is done by combing and holding the hair in the opposite way to which it has been cut. Hair cut vertically is checked horizontally, and hair cut horizontally is checked vertically. Any unevenness in the cut is clearly seen and can be corrected.

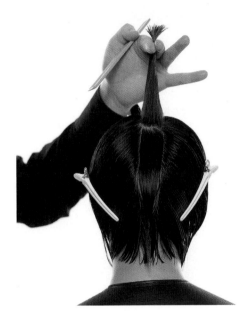

Cross-checking

One-length styles are checked by taking small, equal meshes of hair from either side of the head and at the same time sliding fingers down the length. A balanced one-length haircut is achieved when the fingers reach the ends at the same time (see step 3 on page 168).

Layered cuts have an inside/internal shape and are checked for balance by holding meshes of hair at both sides of the head and gliding the fingers from roots to points, checking the weight of the hair and its length. Any unbalanced areas can then be removed. When a haircut is balanced (the same length either side), it is called symmetrical; when a haircut is designed with one side longer than the other, it is called asymmetrical.

Time interval between cuts

Frequent cutting of hair ends is necessary to maintain healthy hair.

Hair ends should be removed by trimming every six to eight weeks; this maintains the hair's best possible condition and manageability, and even hair that is being grown for length should have its split ends removed.

Hair grows at varied rates on different places on the head, so a haircut can easily get out of shape within a few weeks. A very short haircut may therefore need to be tidied up every four weeks.

1 When is it better to cut dry hair?

2 What must you remember about the finished hair length when cutting wet hair?

3 Should hair be cut wet or dry when looking for the natural fall?

4 What safety considerations should you take into account when cutting hair?

5 Why must sharps be disposed of safely?

6 How should cutting tools be kept clean and sterile?

7 How should you check that your clippers are safe to use?

8 The following are all cutting techniques:

- club cutting
- taper cutting
- pointing and texturising
- scissor/clipper over comb
- thinning.

Describe the different tools needed for each technique, the type of effect produced, and state whether the hair should be cut wet or dry.

9 Why is it important to consult with the client throughout the cutting process?

10 Describe the different cutting angles and how they can be used to achieve a variety of layered looks.

11 Explain the importance of keeping the right degree of tension when cutting.

Chapter 8 Men's haircutting

After working through this chapter you will be able to:

- Maintain effective and safe methods of working
- Cut and finish hair to achieve a variety of looks
- Cut beards and moustaches to maintain their shape.

This chapter covers the following NVQ Level 2 units:
Cut Hair Using Basic Techniques

Introduction

Men's barbering includes being able to cut different short layered looks (including various neckline shapes), and being able to cut beards, moustaches and sideburns into shape.

TO DO

Read Chapter 7 and test your knowledge of cutting before reading this chapter. Pay particular attention to the 'To do' sections.

Short layered looks

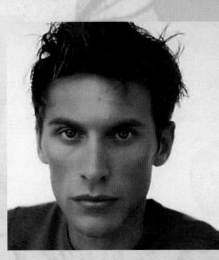

Short layered look

Technically, a man's haircut does not need to match perfectly in the way that a woman's haircut does. It is judged visually, i.e. the finished outline shape must look perfect.

Head analysis

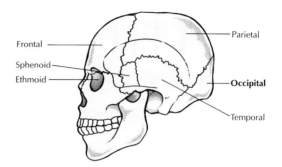

The bones of the head

Head shapes

A man's **occipital bone** tends to be flatter than a woman's occipital bone. Therefore, when you make your **analysis** before cutting, take the weight line below the occipital bone to make sure that the hair doesn't stick out.

Face shapes

Square faces do not suit hard, sharp lines – use a finer graduation around the edges of the haircut for softness.

Round, softer faces can take hard, sharp lines around the edges.

Hair growth patterns

Double crown

Never cut hair too short on a double crown: it will stick up on end!

Neckline shapes

A nape whorl may be tapered into the back neckline, i.e. with no line cut around the bottom neckline.

Back hairlines

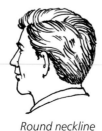

Nape whorl

Normal hairlines that grow down may be cut either square or round by using the scissors or the clippers turned over, depending on the client's requirements. Generally, an uneven hairline is best left longer so that the hair can be cut evenly around it.

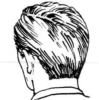

Round neckline

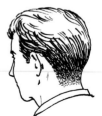

Square neckline

Tapered neckline

Front hairlines

Cowlicks are better left longer and styled the way the hair grows.

Thinning hair and hair loss

Hair loss is caused by the male hormone androgen, which restricts the growth of hair, creating thinning on the front and top of the scalp. The hairs become finer and shorter in length, leaving more of the scalp visible than before.

Male pattern baldness is also a condition that is hereditary. This common form of hair loss begins either at the front temples, receding towards the crown and back or it can begin with hair becoming thin or lost at the crown area.

This type of hair loss is not continuous – the telogen stage is not replaced by the anagen 1 stage – so the thinning or loss of hair is a gradual process.

Male pattern baldness or receding hairlines generally suit a shorter haircut, rather than having a long piece of hair trailing over the top – but use good communication skills here before cutting it off – the client may like it.

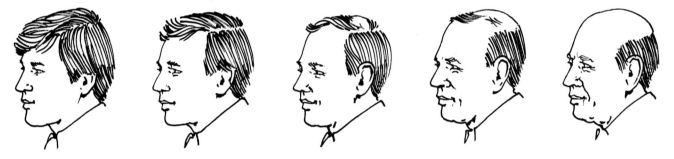

Cicatrical alopecia or scarring, where the hair does not grow, should not be exposed – leave the hair longer to cover over.

The progression of male pattern baldness

Limitations

Hair structure

Straight fine hair must be cut carefully during scissors over comb work especially, or 'steps' will appear. Always keep the comb and scissors moving up and out (away from the head). If you have to remove a step, try **chipping-in** or pointing into it with the tips of your scissors to remove the line.

Wavy or tight, curly hair is best club cut to reduce the curl. Short, African Caribbean hair is best cut out freehand with scissors or clippers (without a guard, which could become entangled in the hair).

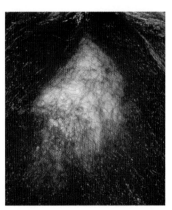

Cicatrical alopecia

REMEMBER
Always check for the presence of added hairpieces, such as a toupée, before you start cutting.

Cutting tight, curly African Caribbean hair

African Caribbean hair that has been permed or straightened needs the same cutting techniques as straight, wavy or curly hair. However, naturally tight, curly African Caribbean hair needs different considerations.

- Always cut it dry, after shampooing and natural drying to achieve a perfect shape.
- Use a wide-toothed afro comb to lift it out from the head and remove any tangles.
- Spray the hair lightly with a thin film of oil from an instant moisturising spray to make it easier to comb through.
- Use freehand cutting – do not hold the hair with your fingers. Allow the hair to fall naturally, then cut with scissors or clippers.
- Keep lifting the hair with the afro comb to check the shape and balance of the style.

REMEMBER

Wet, tight, curly hair will spring back and become much shorter than expected, which is why it is better to cut it dry.

TO DO

Re-read the table on cutting tools and techniques on page 164 in Chapter 7. Ask your supervisor to test you orally on which tools are used on wet and which on dry hair.

Hair texture

Coarse hair may need to be thinned, razored, tapered or texturised to decrease its weight and to achieve the correct shape.

Fine hair needs to be club or blunt cut to increase its weight and make it appear thicker.

Body build

If the client is very tall, don't crop the hair too short or cut a flat-top. Leave some weight in the hair to balance the body.

Cutting tools

Health and safety in barbering

- Clippers must be sterilised before using for each client. If the clipper has cut the skin, the blades must be removed and cleaned and sterilised.
- Hands must be cleaned before each client.
- Skin disorders and cuts must be covered with a suitable waterproof dressing.
- All tools and equipment must be disinfected or sterilised after each client.

TO DO

- Re-read Chapter 3 regarding sterilisation of tools and equipment.
- List and describe four methods of sterilisation.

Scissors

Most hairdressers use $4\frac{1}{2}$ to 5 inch scissors for cutting women's hair, and use only half an inch of the blade for cutting. Men's haircuts often take about 20 minutes, and therefore you need longer blades ($5\frac{1}{2}$ to 6 inches) to cut more quickly.

Thinning scissors are used for blending in weight lines and for softening hard lines, by being inserted at the ends of the hair.

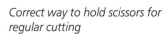
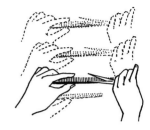

Correct way to hold scissors for regular cutting

TO DO

Practise holding your scissors and opening and closing the top blade with the back of your hand towards you. This is the only way you can cut the hair short enough during barbering.

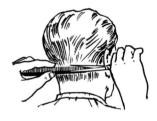

Turning the comb upwards

Combs

Cutting combs are normally used for cutting most hair, but thin flexible barber's combs are needed to cut around the ears and neckline for really short cuts.

Brushes

Close-set bristle brushes are suitable for short, graduated styles as the bristles can pick up the different hair lengths and produce a smooth finished style. Wide-set brushes, e.g. vent brushes produce broken, textured hairstyles.

Using scissors and comb

Clippers

Electric clippers are used extensively for men's barbering techniques and so need to be kept clean and well maintained. The clipper blades need to be oiled or sprayed with clipper oil (this is an antiseptic oil) between clients, and must be kept free of cut hairs. If clippers pull hair, try cleaning and adjusting them.

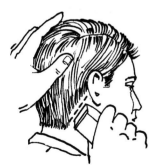

Outlining right side of neck

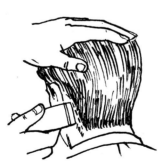

Outlining left side of neck

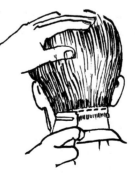

To produce a square nape line, turn clipper over on its cutting edge

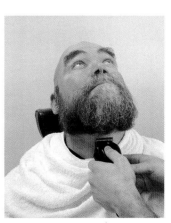

Outlining a beard

REMEMBER

Health and safety
The bottom, static blade of the clippers should always be further forward than the top, moving blade. If the top blade comes too far forward you could cut someone's skin, so be extra careful when clippers are turned over for lining out. Always put on the blade guard when clippers are not in use.

Safety razors

Open razors with disposable blades are used for hairline shaping (lining out) and removing unwanted hair outside the desired outline shape. The best way to do this is to use a piece of cotton wool with warm water and shampoo to soften the hairs first, then stretch the skin tight before removing the hairs with the razor.

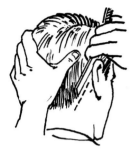

Shave outline below ear

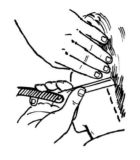

Shave left side of neck using backhand stroke

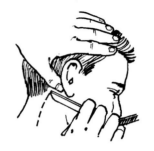

Clean neck below ear

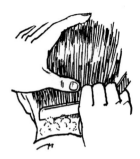

To achieve a square or precision hairstyle, shaving or precision outline is needed

> **TO DO**
> *Ask your supervisor for the salon's policy on how to dispose of used disposable razor blades (sharps). Remember, they are very dangerous pieces of equipment.*

Nozzles

Nozzle attachments for hairdryers are always used for drying men's hair because they concentrate and direct the air flow on to the small section of short hair.

> **TO DO**
> - *Read the Electricity at Work Regulations and the section on using electrical equipment safely in Chapter 3.*
> - *State your responsibilities under the regulations.*

Safety razor

Neck brushes

These are used continually during cutting men's hair, not just at the end of the haircut, to constantly remove the tiny pieces of cut hair that would otherwise stick to the face or neck.

Preparing the client

Gowning up

Gowning up correctly is as important for male clients as it is for women. Cutting collars are particularly useful, especially when a strip of cotton wool is inserted between them and the client's neckline, to prevent hairs from falling down the client's neck.

Positioning yourself

Make sure that you are the correct height for the client. If a hydraulic chair is used, pump it up or lower it to the correct working position before you start. If you are too tall for the client and you have to bend down, bend from the knees, keeping your back straight and working at a 90° angle to the client.

Positioning your client

Make sure that the client is sitting level (without his legs crossed) and that you are working to his natural head position (he must not be reading a book).

Preparing the hair

Before starting a cut it is important to remove any hair dressing products on the hair by loosening with a comb then shampooing. It will also allow for the natural hair fall to be seen clearly.

If the client does not want his hair washed and wet cutting techniques such as razor cutting are required, then spray the hair with warm water from a water spray.

Be aware that if the hair is just wetted with water some styling products may reactivate, making it difficult to control the hair, giving an incorrect cutting result. It can also cause discomfort to the client when combing through as the hair is stuck together.

Confirming the style

Once you have considered all the critical influencing factors (head and face shape, hair growth pattern and hair limitations), then you must confirm both the style and the length of the style with the client.

REMEMBER

Always use your style book to confirm your ideas with your client.

Cutting short, layered looks

Scissor over comb and clipper over comb

Method
Sub-divide the head so that you can work on one area at a time. It is easiest to do the back first, then each side, and lastly the top and front.

The back
- Start with your weight line, cutting it horizontally to the required length. You may then work either down from the weight line to the neckline or from the neckline up to the weight line.
- Removing a little hair at a time, always keep your scissor over comb or clipper over comb work moving.
- The angle of your comb (which is always underneath your scissors or clippers) must be at the same angle as the head and parallel to it. The comb is always moved up and out away from the head, so that the hair will join up with the weight line.

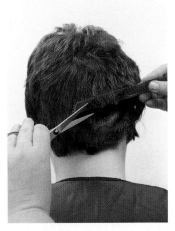

Scissor over comb

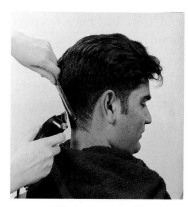

TO DO

Read the section on page 187 on the maintenance of clippers.

REMEMBER

Men's short hair dries quickly and it is easier to scissor or clipper-over-comb dry hair.

REMEMBER

When you are using a pair of clippers with a guard the guard will follow the head shape as it rests on the scalp while cutting. Therefore, if your client has an uneven head shape (e.g. a flat crown area) then the haircut will also be uneven. This is why many salons will not allow clipper guards to be used.

- Start with a larger comb to cut your weight line and change to your finer barber's comb for the short underneath hair.

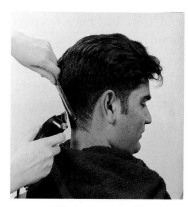

Clipper-over-comb

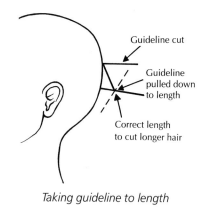

Taking guideline to length

- Always take your cut guideline to your new length of hair to be cut (not the other way around). This is sometimes called a travelling guide.
- You can alter the closeness of a clipper cut by adjusting the blades (normally by flicking a small switch on the side) to vary between $\frac{1}{20}$ mm for the closest to 3 mm for the longest.
- Clipper guards may also be used to vary the length of the cut. The sizes are:

  1   or $\frac{1}{16}$ inch (the shortest)

  2   or $\frac{1}{8}$ inch

  3   or $\frac{1}{4}$ inch

  4   or $\frac{3}{8}$ inch (longer hair)

                 $\frac{1}{2}$ inch

                 1 inch

  depending on the manufacturer.

- When you are cutting very short necklines clipper across the head to cross-check the cut as hair grows in all directions. If the hair grows upwards you will need to clipper the hair down in the opposite direction.
- An undercut style is where the hair is clippered off underneath and either layered or all one length on top. Section off the longer hair first, then clipper off the underneath hair before cutting the top hair to shape.

Fading

Fading is a term that is often used in African Caribbean barbering and describes a type of tapering that goes into the haircut, sometimes as far as the crown.

Other layering techniques

Layering techniques may also be adopted for styles:

- with a parting
- with a fringe
- where the ears are exposed or when the ears are covered

to include natural hair growth patterns such as a double crown or cowlick.

REMEMBER

Whatever style you are cutting look at the natural fall and hairline at all times – you cannot cover over mistakes easily on a man's short haircut.

Styles without a parting

These may be worn:

- back off the face
- forwards on to the face
- brushed across to either side.

The cutting is always the same on top – i.e. it is held at 90° and perfectly even when checked in every direction.

REMEMBER

Always protect the ears during cutting by covering with either your comb or your hand.

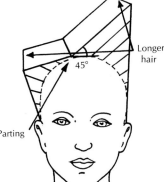

Hair cut without a parting

Styles with a parting

These normally have longer hair on either side of the parting to weigh the hair down. The hair is over-directed and held at 45°, not 90°, to create the length. The longer length weight line is created first and then the shorter layers are held at 45° and blended in to match.

Styles without a fringe

In these styles the hair is worn either back off the face or over to the side.

Styles with a fringe

These are when the hair is styled forward on to the face. To cut the hair with or without a fringe the front hair may be the same length as the top or a little longer, but still matching the layers.

The longer front hair is needed for blow drying back into a 'quiff' or 1950s style, or if the fringe needs to cover a high forehead. Always texturise or 'chip into' (chipping is the same as pointing) the ends of a fringe to create softness on a man's haircut.

Styles with ears exposed

In such styles the hair is cut around the ear against the natural hairline. Always look at the distance between this hairline and the ears – there should not be a large gap or space. If the natural hairline is higher than the ears leave the hair a little longer to reduce the gap. Check the length of the sides with your client – does he want sideburns, a straight line or a pointed shape?

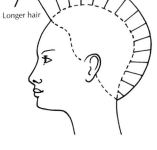

Hair cut with a parting

Hair left longer at the front of a fringe or quiff

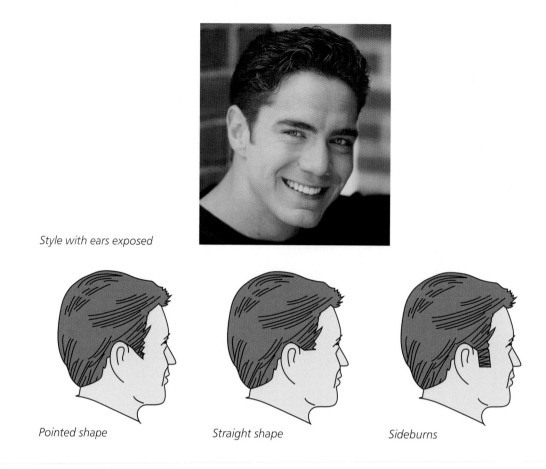

Style with ears exposed

Pointed shape   *Straight shape*   *Sideburns*

Once you have created the shape you may have to remove any unwanted hair with an open razor. Remember to check in the mirror to see that the sideburns are level at both sides.

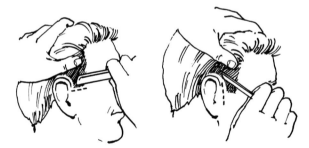

Shaving sideburn to proper length   *Shave over ear*

Styles where the ears are covered

These also need careful cutting. Never pull the hair tight or use tension over the ears because the hair will lift up and become shorter when you let go! Just comb the hair evenly and cut it freehand to achieve the correct length.

Completing the cut

Cross-checking a man's haircut

The difference between checking a man's haircut and checking a woman's haircut is that you should only cross-check a man's cut vertically. You do not cut the corners off as you would for a woman's cut. The result should be more square than round.

To check the shape and balance, look at the man's profile from all angles, not just through the mirror. Place a white towel over your shoulder (unless the hair is white, when you should use a dark towel) to give a clear background and to see the shape properly.

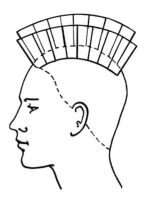

Cross-checking a man's haircut

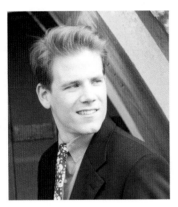

Conventional finish with blow dry lotion

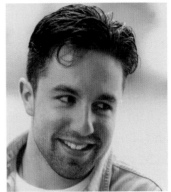

Using light men's cream for a soft finish

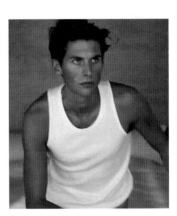

Commercial men's look

Gent's traditional technique

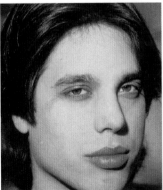

Step 1

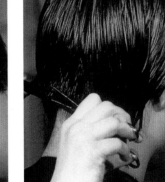

Step 2

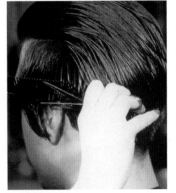

Step 3

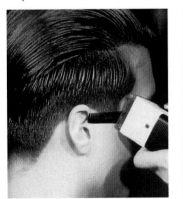

Step 4

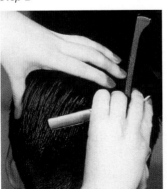

Step 5

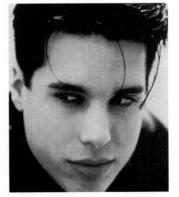

Step 6

Finishing off

Always ask the client if he is satisfied with the result and show him the back of the haircut with the back mirror.

Although you have continually used the neck brush throughout the service, finally check that he is free from all excess hair cuttings once you have finished.

Hair tonics

Also known as friction lotions, hair tonics are used to:

- help correct scalp disorders
- stimulate the scalp
- groom the hair.

The tonic should only be applied to clean hair, unless stated in the manufacturer's instructions.

Applying hair tonics

- Protect the client as per salon requirements.
- Shampoo and condition hair as required and towel dry the hair.
- Apply lotion by sprinkling, being careful not to allow lotion to drip on to the skin or the wet hair to touch the face.
- Massage the lotion into the scalp using friction massage (see page 113).
- Comb hair into desired style.

Styling products

If you are drying off the hair and need more control, use an even distribution of a light blow dry spray.

Once the hair is dry you can give a final shine or polish by using:

- dressing cream (which is lighter than wax) for fine, light-coloured hair
- wax for darker, heavier hair.

REMEMBER

Show the client how much styling product to use on his hair. Many clients use too much and often suffer from flaking scalps.

TO DO

Check with your supervisor and find out how long it should take you to cut a short graduated cut with:
- *clippers*
- *scissors over comb.*

TEST YOUR KNOWLEDGE

1 Describe the differences between cutting techniques and layering techniques and how they can be used to achieve a variety of layered looks.
2 List the cutting techniques that should be used on wet hair and the ones that should be used on dry hair.
3 Why is it important to cut to the natural hairline in men's hairdressing?
4 Describe how to maintain clippers.

Cutting men's facial hair

Men's facial hair can enhance the wearer's appearance by apparently altering the shape of the face – it can make a long face appear narrower, or completely disguise a receding chin.

Fashions and trends in beards, moustaches and sideburns change rapidly, although some cultures, such as Sikhs and Orthodox Jews, have very strict rules as to how facial hair should be worn.

Here are some examples of the many different types that have been worn in the past and some that are still worn today.

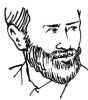
Medium full beard

Balbo beard

Modern beards

Goatee beard

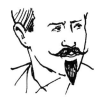
Handlebar and chin puff

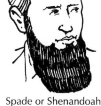
Spade or Shenandoah beard

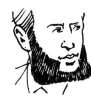
Old Dutch beard

Hulihee beard

Franz Josef beard

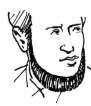
Chin curtain beard

Traditional beards

REMEMBER

A man has to consciously grow a beard. He is making a statement about himself, so cutting facial hair is just as important as cutting scalp hair.
Before you begin to cut, consider your client's reasons for wearing facial hair.

The military

Walrus moustache

Modern moustaches

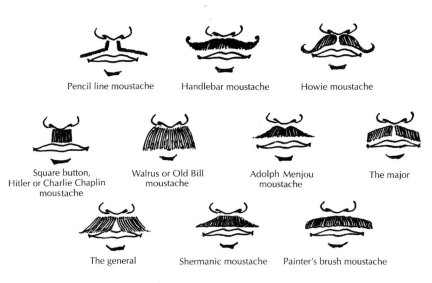

Pencil line moustache Handlebar moustache Howie moustache

Square button,
Hitler or Charlie Chaplin
moustache Walrus or Old Bill
moustache Adolph Menjou
moustache The major

The general Shermanic moustache Painter's brush moustache

Traditional moustaches

TO DO

- *Research the latest magazines and journals for illustrations of current beard and moustache shapes.*
- *Add these to your style book.*

Head and face shapes

- The oval face shape is ideal and suits any style.
- For round and square face shapes beards need to be styled to reduce the width and to be cut flatter at the sides.
- The long face shape needs to be made to appear shorter and wider. A moustache will help this.
- A beard will help to cover and minimise a small or receding chin.
- Sideburns may be part of the facial or scalp hair, or blend with both. (Sideburn shaping has been described on page 192.)

Natural growth patterns

Facial hair grows in certain directions in the same way that scalp hair does. It mostly grows downwards and outwards, and occasionally grows in circular shapes under the chin.

TO DO

Check with your supervisor to see if your salon has any particular requirements for gowning up when cutting men's facial hair.

REMEMBER

The shape of beards, moustaches or sideburns should always blend with and balance the hairstyle – consult with your client before starting. Generally, a client with heavy features will need large facial hair designs, and a client with fine, small facial features will need smaller facial hair designs.

Hair structures and textures

Examine the hair carefully – it may be straight or curly, coarse or fine, dense or sparse and will need cutting accordingly. Facial or beard hair is generally wavy or curly and much stronger and coarser than scalp hair.

Look at the distribution of the facial hair – there may be too much, e.g. a great deal of hair on the neck area, which needs to be removed.

Or there may be too little – e.g. a scarred area or facial alopecia, having no hair growth and this can be seen when it is cut short (by which time it is too late).

TO DO

Re-read the section about client consultation in Chapter 1, complete your consultation sheet and confirm the beard/moustache shape with the client by the use of photographs. Check the outcome of your consultation with your supervisor.

Preparation

TO DO

- *Re-read the section in Chapter 1 on abnormal hair and scalp conditions.*
- *List and describe the effects of dealing with the non-infectious and infectious skin conditions that must be considered before cutting facial hair.*

Gowning up

The client's clothes must be protected as normal, and both of his eyes need to be covered with a feathered-out strip of neck wool.

A towel should be placed diagonally across the client's chest and one side tucked into the collar. The opposite corner of the towel is then folded diagonally over the top and tucked into the other side of the collar. There should be no gap between the client's neck and the towel.

The outline shape of the facial hair must be perfectly balanced and symmetrical when complete. It is sometimes difficult to see this shape if the background is the same colour as his hair. Therefore, try to use a light-coloured gown or towel for dark beards, and darker gowns or towels for lighter beards.

Positioning your client

You will need to work with your client in a reclined position by adjusting the barber's chair and head rest. (If you don't have a barber's chair, recline the client at the back wash-basin and place a towel under his neck for comfort.)

TO DO

Practise adjusting the barber's chair in all its different heights and positions – before you take your first client.

REMEMBER

When you are cutting beard or facial hair the clippings are very sharp and can be dangerous to skin and eyes. Always protect your client as much as possible – and ask him to keep his eyes closed during cutting if they are not covered.

Cutting tools

The tools used for cutting moustaches and beards are often lighter and smaller than usual. This is for precision and accuracy when you are working with delicate shapes and patterns in small areas.

Disentangling

Disentangle the beard by combing it downwards with a wide-toothed comb.

Cutting methods

Scissor over comb

Using small sections, start in the centre of the chin and work out towards the right side and then the left side. Always keep the comb and scissors moving. The closer your comb is held to the face the shorter the cut will be.

TO DO

● Re-read the section in Chapter 3 on the sterilisation of tools and equipment.

● List and describe four methods of each.

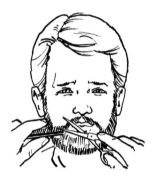

Trimming moustache and beard

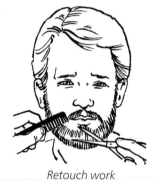

Retouch work

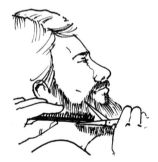

Trimming excess hair

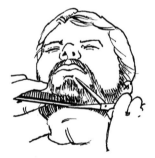

Tapering and blending the beard

Cutting a beard with scissors

Clipper over comb

Cordless or rechargeable clippers are much easier to use for facial hair because you are continually twisting and turning the clippers during cutting. Clipper guards are useful for short beards but may become entangled in longer ones. The final shape may be outlined with clippers.

Clippers with adjustable blades have a lever or a switch, which will either increase or decrease the space between the moving and still-cutting blades. The smaller the gap between the blades the closer the cut will be to the skin.

Clippers must be kept clean from hair cuttings and regularly oiled with professional clipper oil. Clipper oil is a very thin natural oil, which does not evaporate or slow down the power of the clippers. A few drops must be placed between the blades every few haircuts.

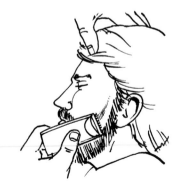

Outlining the upper part of the beard

To clean the blades thoroughly you need to loosen the screws beneath the blades to free them. Loose cut hairs can then be brushed out and cleaned away.

When you put the blades back together you must realign them so that they don't cut too close or allow the moving blade to touch the skin.

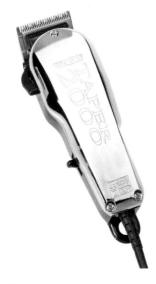

Extreme right-hand tooth of top blade must be touching the big tooth on the bottom blade

End of top blade teeth should be 1/32" to 1/16", 0.79 mm to 1.59 mm, back from bottom blade. This is important so that the clipper doesn't cut too close or allow the moving blade to touch the skin

Extreme left-hand tooth of top blade must be covering, or be to the left of, the first small tooth of bottom blade

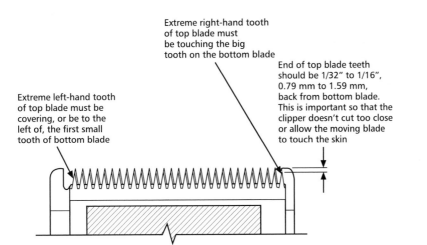

Clipper blades

Clipper

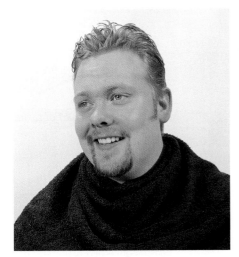

Tidying up a beard: Step 1

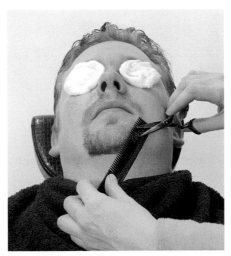

Step 2

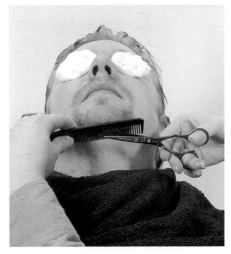

Step 3

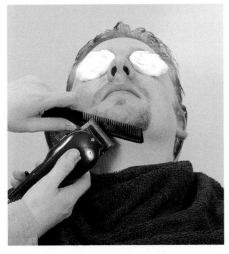

Step 4

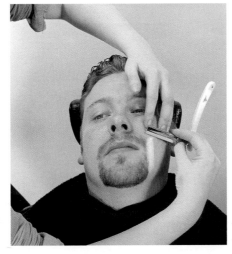

Step 5

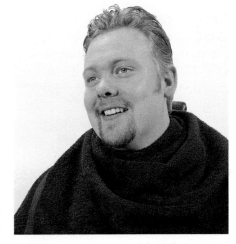

Step 6

Freehand cutting

The outlines of beards or moustaches are usually done freehand, without holding the hair in place with a comb or your fingers. Always support your scissors with your first finger when cutting a moustache to protect the client's lips.

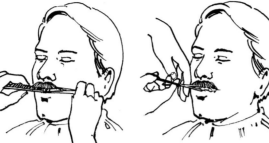

Thinning the moustache   *Trimming the moustache*

TO DO

Check with your supervisor and find out how long it should take you to:
- *cut a beard*
- *cut a moustache.*

Moustache trimming

Razoring

A disposable open razor can be used in the same way as lining out to remove any unwanted hair outside the desired shape.

TO DO
- *Re-read the section in Chapter 3 on the safety aspects of using razors and clippers.*
- *Find out your local by-law requirements for barbering services.*

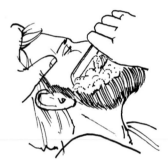

Shaving unwanted part of beard

Finishing off

Remove all the beard clippings from your client with your neck brush then ask the client if he is satisfied with the result as you show him in the mirror.

TO DO
- *Read the health and safety regulations on page 61 on the disposal of waste materials.*
- *Ask your supervisor if this is the procedure used in your salon.*

REMEMBER

Accidents can happen – re-read the section on page 180 concerned with cutting yourself or the client in the salon. You are more likely to cut the client during barbering than when you are working on a female client. Use alum powder on a small piece of damp cotton wool to stop any bleeding, and ask the client to hold it on to the cut.

TEST YOUR KNOWLEDGE

1 Why is it important to match beard shapes with the client's facial characteristics?

2 Why is it important to consult with your client before cutting his facial hair?

3 Describe the health and safety requirements regarding the use of cutting equipment.

4 Describe the difference between adjusting and aligning clippers.

5 Describe your responsibilities under the Electricity at Work Regulations 1992.

6 What should you do if you accidentally cut your own skin?

7 What should you do if you accidentally cut your client's skin?

8 What particular safety considerations must be taken into account when cutting facial hair?

9 How should you dispose of used razor blades?

Chapter 9 Perming, relaxing and neutralising

After working through this chapter you will be able to:

- Choose and use the correct products, tools and techniques
- Perm and neutralise hair using three basic techniques
- Understand the differences between Caucasian, African Caribbean and Asian hair types for relaxing and perming
- Relax hair
- Resolve any problems.

This chapter covers the following NVQ Level 2 units:
Perm and Neutralise Hair Using Basic Techniques
Perm, Relax and Neutralise Hair
Perm, Relax and Neutralise African Caribbean Hair

Permanent waving and relaxing are techniques used to change the shape of the hair permanently. As the hair continues to grow, its natural shape may be seen at the roots or **regrowth** area.

Client consultation for perming or relaxing

A good perm or relaxer depends not only on your practical skills but also on your ability to make the right decisions about your client's hair, both before and during perming or relaxing. Always confirm the desired effect with your client before you start work.

Perming

Always regard a permanent wave or relaxer as an on going process, which means that you must keep your mind on the job at all times to make sure things are going the way you want them to.

Gowning up

Gown up the client with a protective gown, cape and towels to protect from perm and neutraliser lotions, both of which can damage clothes and skin.

Cutting

Most hair needs some cutting, to remove any perm on the ends, to remove dry brittle ends or simply to reshape before perming. Some hairdressers prefer to cut before perming, while others cut the hair after perming and before styling. It is up to you and your client to decide, but remember: hair always appears shorter after perming as the curl lifts the hair up.

Perming tests

Always check the scalp for cuts and abrasions before perming as the chemicals can affect these very severely. Small cuts and abrasions can be protected with collodian (New-Skin).

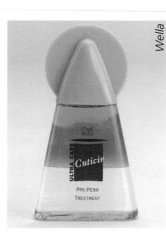

Wella

Pre-perm treatment

Perming coloured and bleached hair

Hair that has been permanently coloured or bleached is more porous and will absorb perm lotion very quickly. You must, therefore, choose a strength of lotion especially for this type of hair (often No. 2, 3 or 4 strength), also refer to the manufacturer's instructions.

Pre-perm treatments

These treatments are used to even out the hair's porosity along its length to achieve even curl results and to prevent over-processed ends.

Some hair is unevenly porous (e.g. very dry ends) and a pre-perm treatment will need to be applied to those areas of hair. Pre-perm lotions are applied to towel-dried hair and left on; they are not rinsed out before perming.

Explaining costs

The client will want to know why some perm lotions cost more than others, so you will have to be able to explain the benefits of each. Here are some possible reasons why some products are more expensive.

- It is a good, strong lotion and will last.

- It contains special conditioning agents to keep hair shiny.
- It is a type of acid perm, which breaks down fewer bonds in the hair during processing and so does less damage.

The chemical process of perming

You will need to understand the chemical process so you are able to select the correct type of lotion for your client's hair.

There are three stages in perming:
1 softening – the hair is softened by the perm lotion
2 moulding – the lotion causes the hair to take up its new shape while it is wound around the perm rods
3 fixing – the hair is fixed permanently into its new shape using neutraliser.

TO DO
Re-read the section in Chapter 1 on hair structure, especially the cuticle and the cortex, and make notes of the differences between the temporary and the permanent bonds.

Softening and moulding the hair during perming
The strong disulphide bonds in the hair are made of an amino acid called **cystine** – these are the bonds that are broken by the perm lotion during the perming process. These bonds are broken because alkaline perm lotions contain a reducing agent called **ammonium thioglycollate** (you can smell the ammonia when you open the bottle). As the perm lotion soaks through the cuticle scales and enters the cortex, the reducing agent adds hydrogen to the disulphide bonds, to form a new amino acid, **cysteine**. The hair is now softened and will mould itself to the shape of the perm rods.

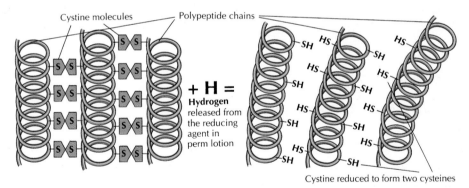

Softening and moulding the hair

TO DO
Re-read the section in Chapter 5 on the pH scale, and make notes on the effect of acids and alkalis on the hair.

Choosing an acid or an alkaline perm

Alkaline perms
These have a pH of approximately 9.5, which opens up the cuticle scales, make the hair more porous, and allows the perm lotion to enter the cortex.

The higher the perm lotion's pH, the more damaging it is to the hair.

This is why conditioning agents are added to alkaline perms – and why acid perms are becoming increasingly popular. However, alkaline perms are the usual choice for both normal and virgin hair.

The benefits of alkaline perms:
- strong curl pattern
- fast **processing time**
- room temperature processing.

Alkaline perms should be used when:
- hair is resistant
- a tight, strong curl movement is required
- the client has a history of early curl relaxation.

Acid perms

These have activators added to them and rely on heat to open up the cuticle scales so that they can penetrate the cortex. They generally have a slightly acid pH (5.5–7) and contain a chemical called glyceryl monothioglycollate.

Fewer bonds in the hair are broken by acid perms, which is why they are said to be better for use on fragile, damaged hair and hair that is easy to process.

The benefits of acid/lower pH perms:
- soft curl pattern
- slower, more controllable processing time
- gentler treatment for delicate hair types.

Acid/lower pH perms should be used when:
- perming delicate or fragile hair, i.e. colour-treated hair
- a soft, more natural curl movement is required
- style support is required more than a strong curl.

Matching hair type to perm lotion

TO DO

Find out:
- *what perm lotions your salon has to offer*
- *how many strengths are available*
- *the price of each.*

Perm lotions are made for many different types of hair:
- resistant – non-porous, fine hair which often dries very quickly, or some types of coarse white hair
- normal – virgin hair that has not been treated with chemicals
- tinted – hair that has been processed with permanent tints
- bleached – hair that has been processed with bleach (including highlights)
- over-porous – hair that is in a very dry, porous condition.

Hair that is generally more porous needs a weaker perm lotion and resistant hair needs a stronger perm lotion. For example, a normal-strength alkaline lotion on fine, fragile, porous hair would break too many bonds, breaking the hair and making it dry, dull, brittle and possibly frizzy. A normal-strength acid lotion used on long, coarse hair would not break enough bonds, giving very little curl – and the perm would tend to drop.

Perming equipment

Perm rods
Many types of perm rods are available. The most common ones have rubber bands for fastening, but Molten permers are also frequently used.

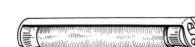

Perm rod fastened

Rods are available in many sizes and are colour-coded so that the sizes can be easily recognised.

Always wash, rinse and dry perm rods after use. Use a little talcum powder on the rubbers after drying to stop them from perishing.

Pin-tail comb
The metal pin-tail end of the comb is ideal for sectioning during perm winding and woven highlights, but extreme care must be taken when using this comb due to its pointed end.

End papers
These are specially designed, absorbent papers that make winding easier and help to prevent 'fishhooks' or buckled ends.

Barrier creams
Barrier creams are thick, heavy, protective creams that should be applied to the client's hairline if they are sensitive to perm lotion. The cream acts as a barrier.

Always use barrier cream or Petroleum jelly before relaxing hair – the chemicals are very strong and can burn both skin and scalp.

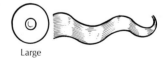
Large

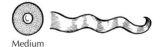
Medium

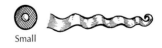
Small

Effect of different rod sizes

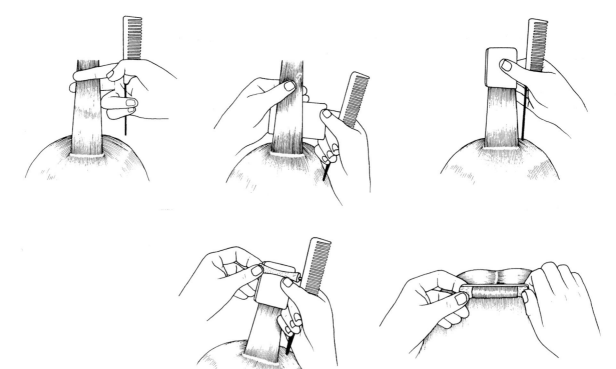

Applying end papers

Cotton wool

Cotton wool strips must be pre-dampened with warm water to prevent perm lotion (and neutraliser) being absorbed into the skin during use. Place them around the client's hairline to prevent any lotion from running into their eyes, ears or neck. If the cotton wool has absorbed any lotion during processing, replace it immediately to prevent skin burns.

Cotton wool can be used to absorb excess moisture from the curlers before the neutraliser is applied.

REMEMBER

Good preparation saves time and inconvenience and looks professional.

Protective gloves

These should always be worn when applying perm lotion and neutraliser to prevent skin damage. If they are difficult to put on because your hands are damp, sprinkle some talcum powder inside them.

A protective apron should also be worn to protect your clothes as both perm lotion and neutraliser will stain them on contact.

See page 62 for your responsibilities under the Personal Protective Equipment at Work Regulations 1992.

TO DO

- Have a look at pages 205–207 on the preparation of equipment to check that you have not forgotten anything.
- For ease of use keep your trolley on your right side if you are right-handed (left side if you are left-handed), and avoid any obstructions.
- Re-read the section in Chapter 3 on the sterilisation of tools and equipment.
- List and describe four methods of each.

Perm caps

Plastic caps are used on the client's hair during processing. They aid development by containing the client's body heat.

Accelerators and hood dryers

Many perm lotions need extra heat to make them work. Use either a hood dryer (with a perm cap) or an accelerator in these cases.

TO DO

Check the manufacturer's instructions on all the perm lotions in your salon to see:
- *which perms need heat*
- *which perms need a plastic cap*
- *the recommended development time.*

TEST YOUR KNOWLEDGE

1   Why should you prepare and position your tools and equipment properly before starting to perm or relax hair?

2   Why should you always use personal protective equipment?

3   Why is it important to report shortages of both product stock and sundries to the relevant person?

Perming method

Shampooing

The hair should be shampooed with a plain soapless shampoo that contains no extra additives such as conditioner or medicated ingredients. These additives would act as a barrier or film on the hair, and prevent the perm lotion from entering the hair shaft. For the same reason, it is not normal procedure to use a conditioner before perming (unless you are using a specialist pre-perm product).

Towel drying the hair before perming

Once you have combed the hair thoroughly to remove all tangles you must towel it dry to prevent the perm lotion from becoming diluted. Use a dry towel and gently squeeze the hair between the two sides of the towel.

The hair should be left wet, but not dripping with water. Since hair is absorbent it must be kept slightly damp so that it does not absorb perm lotion too quickly. In case the hair does dry out too much during winding, keep a water spray nearby to dampen it down.

Sectioning

Sectioning is very important when you are learning to perm – it enables you to work quickly and without being muddled, and to see the size of the rods already used.

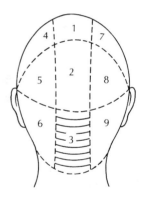

Traditional nine-section method

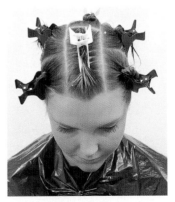

Section 1

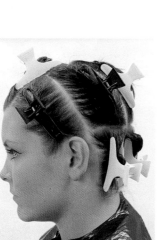

Sections 1, 2, 3 and 4

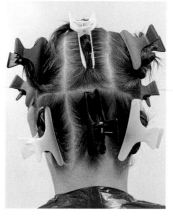

Nine sections

There are many different methods of sectioning but the most common is the traditional nine-section method. This allows you to obtain neat, even sections and prevents mistakes such as root drag.

- Start at the front hairline and make sure that section 1 is in the centre, and parallel. It should end just before the crown area.
- Always measure the size of the sections against the length of the perm rod – the section should be just a little smaller than the rod.
- Secure each section with a section clip or a butterfly clamp, neatly on its own base.
- Continue with section 2, ending level with the top of the ear.
- Now complete section 3 down to the nape.
- Check that sections 1, 2 and 3 are in the centre of the head, not lopsided.
- Continue with section 4, measuring both the top and bottom of the section with the perm rod.
- To complete sections 5 and 6, section from the top of section 3 across to the top of the ear, level with the bottom of section 4.
- Repeat sections 4, 5 and 6 on the opposite side of the head to complete sections 7, 8 and 9.

Sub-sectioning

Sub-sections are the smaller sections taken for each individual perm rod.

The length of the perm rod decides the size of the large section, but the depth or width of the rod dictates the size of the sub-section.

Each sub-section must be parallel, or uneven winding will result.

Once the hair has been sub-sectioned, the hair should be combed smoothly at an angle of 90° away from the head.

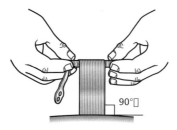

Winding the hair at 90°

The width of the hair sections that should be taken when winding and during the application of treatments and tints is determined by hair density.

Dense, thick hair needs small, fine sections per rod, to prevent a weak curl or patchy application finish.

REMEMBER

Always ask the client to position their head correctly (forwards, upright or sideways) for you so that you can work properly.

Sparse, thin hair can have larger sections. Pulling the hair towards the roller or rod must be prevented, as this can cause distorted hair shapes, or even break the hair.

Winding the curlers

Use a pin-tail comb to wind the ends around the rod, using end papers if necessary to prevent 'fishhooks'.

Always keep the perm rod parallel to the head during winding or it will not sit properly on its base (the sub-section).

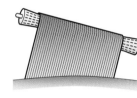
Winding the curlers

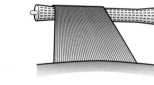
Non-parallel winding

Lopsided winding

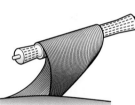
Twisted winding

As clients' heads are round (not square) and the perm rods are straight, perfect winding is difficult to achieve without practice.

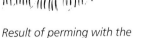
Result of perming with the rubbers fixed too tightly

Winding variations

Directional winding
This is where the hair is wound in the direction of the finished style.

Brick winding
This technique gives a more uniform curl and avoids partings in the finished result.

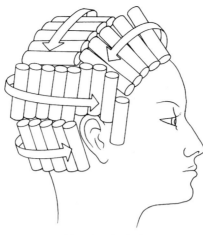

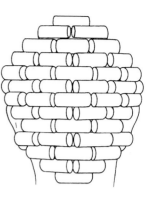

Directional winding

Brick winding

Applying perm lotion

Pre-damping

Pre-damping is when the hair has perm lotion applied *before* winding. This technique is often used for resistant (non-porous) hair or for long hair.

Post-damping

Post-damping is when the lotion is applied *after* winding has been completed, and applicator bottles with special nozzles are often used.

Safety points to remember

● Wear your gloves when applying lotion to the hair.

● Applying lotion can be very dangerous, as it can easily run into the client's eyes. If this does happen, rinse immediately with cold water on a pad of cotton wool until the client says the stinging has stopped.

● Always hold a piece of cotton wool just below the perm rods during lotioning to absorb any excess. A strip of dampened cotton wool around the hairline should always be used to prevent lotion running on to the skin. If any lotion does run on to the skin, the dampened cotton wool must be replaced immediately to prevent the lotion from resting on the skin and burning it.

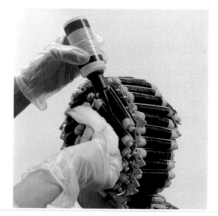

Applying perm lotion

● Pull burns may result if the hair is wound tightly – the neck of the hair follicle opens, allowing perm lotion to enter. If the scalp is scratched this irritation could become infected, causing folliculitis.

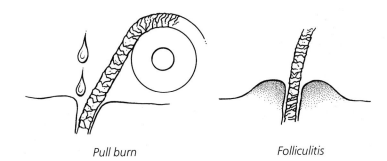

Pull burn   *Folliculitis*

- Many manufacturers' bottles of perm lotion and neutraliser look very similar. To avoid applying the wrong lotion do not get the bottle of neutraliser out until you are ready to neutralise.

Checking curl development 'S' bends

Thin or fine hair normally forms softer wave ridge movements, whereas thick or coarse hair holds a wave ridge movement more easily because it usually has more elasticity. Alkaline perm development produces formed wave movements. Acid perm development produces hair 'stranding' or separation when unwound from the rod and slight wave movement.

Processing and timing the perm

The timing of the moulding stage, where the hair is softened around the perm rods, is crucial. If the lotion is left on too long then the hair will become over-processed, frizzy and will break off.

Over-processed perm

Over-processing can be identified with ease as it cannot keep a good even wave movement due to the lack of elasticity. Once dried the hair feels harsh. Recommended treatments include reconditioning treatments.

Under-processed perm

Under-processing is caused by insufficient processing time. Hair has weak wave movements with unstructured ridges. Hair movement is usually lost after a few shampoo washes.

Even though there is little or no curl or wave movement, you must treat the hair as chemically treated. If hair tests prove satisfactory, then weaker perm lotions must be applied with regular testing or curl formation.

TO DO

Re-read the section in Chapter 1 on development test curls and practise them as often as possible.

The length of time the perm lotion is left on will vary according to:
- the room temperature – heat speeds up chemical reactions, so the hotter the room is the quicker it will work
- the porosity of the hair – the more porous the hair the quicker the reaction
- the client's body heat – if the head is covered with a perm cap, the body heat will be trapped in and the perm will process more quickly

- the strength of the perm lotion – the stronger the perm lotion the quicker it will act
- the pH of the perm lotion – generally the higher the pH, the quicker the reaction
- remember – the neutralising processes will stop any further development of the perm lotion.

Two-stage curly perms

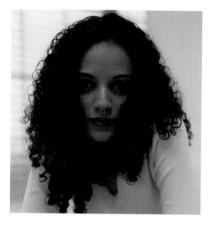

African Caribbean perm

African Caribbean perms, sometimes called 'wet look' or 'curly' perms, are possible on African Caribbean hair because they chemically straighten or relax the curly hair first using a curl rearranger. The hair is then permed with a weaker perm lotion, a curl booster, into larger, softer curls.

Curl rearrangers may be available in three or four different strengths, but curl boosters are available in only one strength.

The method involves relaxing the hair with ammonium thioglycollate using the comb or hands to smooth the hair into a straighter position, then winding the hair on large rods or rollers and applying a liquid gel-based thioglycollate curl booster.

This process is often called reverse perming.

As with all chemical processes, care must be taken not to damage the hair.

Method

- The curl rearranger is applied to the hair after a light pre-perm shampoo if the hair has excess oil, using light massaging movements and tepid water to prevent stimulation of the scalp. The hair is then towel dried. It is preferable that the hair be shampooed at least three days before an African Caribbean perming process to reduce the likelihood of scalp irritation from occuring.
- A pre-conditioning treatment (a protective polymer) is applied to the hair that has been chemically treated. The hair is then covered with a plastic cap and processed under a cool dryer for 10 minutes.
- Always protect the client's skin around the hairline with barrier cream or Petroleum jelly.
- The product is applied in the same way as a tint or a bleach, section by section.
- The hair is then combed straight, gently but firmly.
- The rearranger is then developed according to the manufacturer's directions, taking 10–30 minutes, until the hair becomes less curly, and is smooth, straight, and pliable.

- The hair is thoroughly rinsed then blotted dry with a towel, taking care not to tangle the hair.
- Hair is then wound onto perm rods and a curl booster is applied either before winding (pre-damped) or after winding (post-damped). The curl rearrangers and boosters are thioglycollate chemicals. They swell the hair shaft and break down some of the disulphide bonds.
- The hair is then processed as per the manufacturer's instructions.
- After perm development, the hair is rinsed to remove the curl re-arranger and blotted dry to remove excess moisture.
- Barrier cream and a strip of dampened cotton wool are placed around the hairline. Neutraliser is applied to the rods and timed for development as per manufacturers' instructions.
- After neutralising, the rods are removed and the hair thoroughly rinsed and conditioned.
- A glycerine-based activator/moisturiser is used to define the curls and to achieve a wet look.

REMEMBER

Never perm African Caribbean hair that is badly damaged or has been chemically relaxed. If in doubt, take a pre-perm test curl.

Basing

A petroleum cream product must be applied to the scalp, hairline and ears to protect the skin from the harsh effects of the relaxing product. A cream based product is preferable to petroleum jelly as it melts at a lower temperature easily when applied to the scalp and spreads evenly, giving better coverage and protection by leaving a fine oily film on the skin.

Basing is applied by sectioning the hair into four and then taking fine horizontal sections and applying a thin coat of the basing cream carefully to the scalp.

Relaxing or permanently straightening hair

Relaxers are very popular with clients who have excessively curly or wavy hair because once their hair is permanently straightened they have a much wider choice of hairstyles.

Relaxing hair can also be used to reduce the amount of natural curl in the hair thus making it easier to comb (relax).
Tight, curly African Caribbean hair has more cuticle scales and is initially more difficult to chemically process.

Relaxers work by softening and swelling the hair, breaking the disulphide bonds.

Relaxing creams are extremely alkaline, with a pH of 10–14, which means they are very strong chemicals.
Relaxing products are available in two formulations:
- base formulations require a base (petroleum cream) to be applied
- non-base formulations require no base; this formulation is milder, making it ideal for children.

Previously treated hair must be protected to prevent **overlapping** by applying a cream or oil-based conditioner on to the treated areas up to the **demarcation** line.

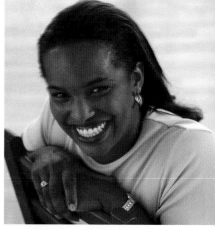

Relaxed hair

TO DO

Re-read the section in Chapter 1 on African Caribbean hair structure.

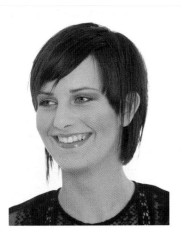

TO DO

Read page 61 regarding the Cosmetic Products (Safety) Regulations 1989, then compare the strengths of the professional relaxing products in your salon with those sold for retail use.

Relaxing products and equipment

The products required are chemical **hair relaxer** (lye or non-lye based); neutraliser; barrier cream which should be applied to protect the scalp; tint brush; plastic tail comb; butterfly clips; protective gloves; apron; cape and towels.

Conditioner fillers

Conditioner fillers are used before chemically relaxing the hair:

- to protect porous/slightly damaged hair
- to prevent hair being over-processed
- to even out the porosity, allowing even processing along the hair shaft.

The conditioner filler or buffer contains a protein polymer that should be rubbed into the hair, combed through to ensure even coverage and dried using a cool hood dryer to completely dry the hair before applying the relaxing product.

To remove curl

Sodium hydroxide relaxers (caustic soda, sometimes called lye) are the strongest and fastest-acting chemicals.

Lye relaxers contain 5–10 per cent sodium hydroxide, which has a pH of 10–14, therefore the stronger the product the higher (more caustic) pH it has.

Calcium hydroxide (occasionally potassium hydroxide) relaxers (sometimes called no-lye) are not as strong and do not require the scalp to be based with a protective product before application. These relaxers are often available for home use, but they are not as effective as other relaxers. Also, they tend to lighten the colour, causing a reddish tinge, and leave the hair more dry and brittle.

Both of these straightening chemicals permanently change the structure of the hair by changing one-third of the cystine bonds into new **lanthionine bonds** (with one sulphur atom), which keep the hair straight. This process is **stopped** (sometimes known as **hydrolysis**) by a **neutralising shampoo**. The low pH of this shampoo stops any further chemical action.

To remove curl

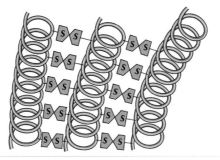

Tight curly/wavy hair with disulphide bonds intact

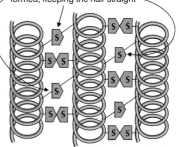

New single sulphur lanthionine bonds formed, keeping the hair straight

After being shaped with straightening cream, processed and having neutralising shampoo added

To reduce the degree of curl

Ammonium thioglycollate, the same chemical that is used to perm hair and make it curly, may also be used to straighten fine, difficult hair, or if the client doesn't want all the curl removed.

These 'thio' straighteners may be either a thick cream, which is used in exactly the same way as the hydroxide relaxers (i.e. the hair is smoothed straight), or normal perm lotion that is combed on to the hair and then wound around large rollers.

Ammonium thioglycollate breaks down the disulphide bonds (by using a reducing agent – hydrogen), and changes the cystine in the hair to cysteine.

Both the cream and liquid processes are stopped by an oxidising neutraliser, which re-forms the broken disulphide bonds and holds the hair in its new shape.

REMEMBER

Never 'steam' hair after using a relaxer – it will revert to being curly.

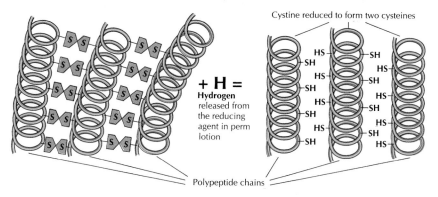

To reduce the degree of curl

Properties of different relaxing chemicals

Sodium hydroxide (lye)

This is a caustic-type hair relaxer that has a softening and a swelling action on hair. The solution penetrates into the cortex layer, breaking the disulphide.

The hair is moulded into shape by the physical action of the comb, brush or hand. The chemical product softens the hair.

There is a high alkaline content to sodium hydroxide, so great care must be taken when it is used as the chemical reaction will take place more quickly on the hair.

Disadvantages of sodium hydroxide:
- unsuitable for Caucasian hair types
- due to the high alkaline pH value, it can cause serious skin and scalp burns.
- hair can discolour if left on too long.

Calcium hydroxide (non-lye)

Disadvantages of calcium hydroxide:
- unsuitable for Caucasian hair
- speed and accuracy of application is needed
- discolouration of the hair can result
- natural hair shine can be reduced with long-term use.

REMEMBER

Sodium and calcium hydroxide relaxers and ammonium thioglycollate straighteners and perms are incompatible – they do not work with each other. All the processed hair must grow out and be cut off before changing from one type of product to the other.

Ammonium thioglycollate

Disadvantages of ammonium thioglycollate:

- using the rearranger as a straightener only can cause serious hair damage due to bonds being broken and not reformed
- does not produce a good straightener result
- slower development and processing than the other chemical straighteners.

Relaxer test

To check the hair's suitability for relaxing:

- take a fine section at the resistant area (usually the nape) and with a small length of foil make a slit across 2 cm from the top and pull the fine hair section through the slit, ensuring the foil is as close to the root as possible
- take another fine hair section at the crown and pull through another foil strip
- apply relaxer to the hair sections and process until relaxed to required straightness, checking every 3–5 minutes.

Note the development time and smoothness required, rinse, apply neutralising shampoo to the section, shampoo the relaxer and towel dry. If the tests prove satisfactory, coat the processed sections with barrier to protect from further damage and process the rest of the hair with relaxer.

If damage occurs, strand test with a milder relaxing product.

REMEMBER

If in doubt choose a weaker product and then apply a stronger product if the process is rather slow.

Matching relaxer to hair type

- Fine, tinted or lightened hair (hair that has previously been chemically treated) – use mild relaxers.
- Normal, medium-textured virgin hair – use regular relaxers.
- Coarse, virgin hair – use strong or super-relaxers.

Heat and relaxers

Heat must never be applied to speed up the process of a relaxing service due to the high pH value of the relaxer; natural body heat will always prove sufficient.

Regrowth

Relaxers should be reapplied every six weeks to two months, depending upon the rate of hair growth.

Regrowth left to grow longer than $\frac{3}{4}$ in (1.5 cm) can cause hair breakage from physical damage due to combing two differently textured hairs on one head; regrowth/virgin hair is coarse and overly curly, so this is combed with more tension through to the processed relaxed hair, which is straight and requires less tension when being combed through. It is combing through these different textures that can break the fragile processed area of the hair.

Precautions

TO DO

Re-read the sections in Chapter 1 on strand tests, elasticity tests, porosity tests and incompatibility tests.

To reduce scalp irritation the hair should not be shampooed for at least three days before the intended service.

Check the following:

- the client's scalp for any soreness, cuts, abrasions or disorders. If in doubt do not proceed – call your supervisor. Leave 72 hours between tinting/bleaching and relaxing treatments
- the client's hair condition for:

  elasticity and **tensile strength** (elasticity test)

  tightness of curl (strand test, i.e. product strength and timing)

  texture and porosity (porosity test)

  previous chemical processes (incompatibility test)

  any breakage (elasticity test)

  If you are in any doubt, proceed with the necessary test and suggest some reconditioning treatments
- the client's record card for any previous treatments
- agree the exact degree of straightness the client requires (use photographs from the style books).

TO DO

Take three cuttings each of tight curly and wavy hair and strand test them with a sodium hydroxide, calcium hydroxide and ammonium thioglycollate relaxer. Make a note of the development times and any differences in the elasticity and condition of the hair.

Points to remember: health and safety

Relaxers are very strong chemicals.

- Make sure that you have sufficient product knowledge. Try writing out the manufacturer's instructions in your own words and checking with your supervisor.
- Carry out a full consultation of the hair and scalp before starting, carrying out the necessary tests, if required.
- Do not relax damaged hair or use excessive heat on relaxed hair.
- Correctly protect the client and always apply protective base cream when using sodium hydroxide products.
- Always wear protective clothing and gloves.
- Do not shampoo the hair immediately prior to sodium hydroxide relaxing.
- Never mix or apply ammonium thioglycollate products with sodium hydroxide products.

REMEMBER

The scalp is very sensitive after either corn row plaits or extensions have been removed. Do not chemically relax hair on the same day that they are removed. To reduce scalp irritation, the hair should be shampooed at least three days before the intended service.

- Do not relax hair that has been previously chemically treated or coloured with metallic tints.
- Always follow the manufacturer's instructions.
- Use professional tools and equipment and wide-toothed combs and avoid scratching the client's scalp.
- Never overlap the product on to previously treated hair.
- If the product touches the scalp or skin for a prolonged period it will cause serious irritation, burning and damage. If the client complains that his or her skin or scalp are 'burning', rinse the relaxer off immediately and use the neutralising shampoo to fix the broken bonds.
- Always use the back wash-basin to remove the relaxer and for applying the neutralising shampoo.
- If the relaxer accidentally enters the eye it could cause blindness, so shield the unaffected eye with one hand, and flush the affected eye with lots of water. Seek medical help if the irritation persists.
- If the product stays in contact with the hair for too long the hair may become brittle, break off or even dissolve. Do not relax the hair if you think there will be any hair breakage.
- Never apply the product to hair that has already been relaxed – apply it only to new regrowth.
- Make sure that you are using the correct straightening chemical for the hair and the correct strength of chemical. If in doubt, check with your supervisor.
- Never use any additional heat (from hairdryers or accelerators or steamers) when processing sodium or calcium hydroxide relaxers – they develop very quickly and could dissolve the hair.
- Always wear rubber gloves and a protective apron, and gown up your client properly.
- Always protect the client's hairline and scalp by applying Petroleum jelly or special basing cream.
- Never mix relaxers, neutralisers and other products from different manufacturers – they are unlikely to work together. If the hair becomes damaged you will be legally responsible.
- Remove all relaxer thoroughly prior to neutralising.
- Condition the hair and scalp before setting and drying.
- Complete all record cards thoroughly.
- Keep record cards up to date.

Method

Gown up as for perming.

Do not shampoo the hair or brush the scalp. Apply the basing cream or Petroleum jelly to the scalp area section by section (like a tint). Place the cream, do not press or rub it in, as it must not cover the hair.

Check the manufacturer's instructions, and wear gloves. If a special conditioner filler (pre-relaxing treatment) needs to be used, apply it evenly at this stage and blot off any excess.

Then follow with either the comb/brush method or the finger method, both described below.

Comb/brush method

For the comb/brush method, transfer some relaxing cream from the tub into a bowl using a spatula. Section the whole head into four and, starting at the right nape section, take $\frac{1}{2}$–1 cm wide sub-sections.

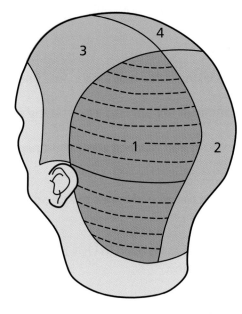

Divide hair into four sections

Start at the nape area, taking section widths of $\frac{1}{2}$–1 cm, depending on the thickness/curliness of the hair.

Apply relaxer cream using the back of a tail comb or brush to the topside, then to the underside, avoiding the scalp area. The back of the comb is normally used for clients with sensitive scalps.

Work up the back quarter sections from nape to crown, then the front quarter sections from crown to front hairline.

Once completed, re-check the sections, applying more relaxer to the hair if the hair has absorbed it all.

Apply relaxer to the front hairline last, as this will be the most porous area.

Gently smoothing the relaxer through the hair spreads the cream and stretches the hair smooth. Do not use excessive pressure when combing.

With previously straightened hair, apply to the regrowth only, taking care not to overlap on to the previously straightened hair.

REMEMBER
The client should remove glasses or contact lenses before the relaxing process.

REMEMBER
You should take no longer than eight minutes to apply a relaxer because these strong chemicals process very quickly.

Hair ends can be protected with cream conditioner or barrier cream during the straightening process.

TO DO

Ask other stylists in your salon if they use any other methods of applying relaxing agents.

Leave the hair as straight as possible. Do not continually comb the hair – it may easily break.

Finger method

This method is used when relaxing virgin hair for the first time.

Transfer some relaxing cream from the tub into a bowl using a spatula.

Section the whole head into four and, starting at the right nape section, take 1 cm wide sections.

Apply cream using the palms of the gloved hands to spread the product and smooth the hair straight.

Work up the back quarter sections from nape to crown, then the front quarter sections from crown to front hairline.

Smooth the hair straight with your gloved hand to spread the product. Once completed, cross-check the application in the opposite direction, applying more relaxer to the hair if the hair has absorbed it all.

Apply relaxer to the front hairline last as this will be the most porous area.

For both methods

Develop the product according to the manufacturer's instructions. This may take 2–18 minutes. Check it continually once applied.

Gently scrape the cream to remove from the hair using the back of a comb, and then gently lift the mesh with the tail end of a comb or brush and check for straightness and smoothness.

If the mesh has a curl wave movement, leave to process, reapplying more cream to the area.

If the mesh is smooth or has the required straightness, then the hair should be rinsed thoroughly to remove the relaxer cream.

TO DO

- Watch your stylist taking a strand test and testing for straightness during relaxing.
- Ask your supervisor if you may be allowed to take a strand test under supervision.
- Check your salon's time allocation for applying a relaxer.

When processing is complete rinse at a back wash-basin with a strong stream of warm water. Remove the cream from the hairline, using your fingers to gently part the hair.

Rinse until the water runs clear. Some manufacturers advise the use of a reconstructing treatment at this stage, which should be left for five minutes before the neutralising shampoo is applied.

Relaxing with sodium hydroxide or calcium hydroxide (retouch)

This process, known as a **retouch**, is carried out in order to relax any new hair growth. The process is the same as that followed for first time application, but the new growth only is processed.

To avoid damage and breakage to the hair a conditioner filler or barrier cream must be applied to all the hair that has been previously processed, up to the demarcation line.

Perming and relaxing faults and corrections

FAULT	CAUSES	CORRECTION
The perm is not curly enough	Poor shampooing (hair greasy) Poor neutralising Too few perm rods used Perm rods too large Perm lotion too weak Not enough perm lotion applied Perm lotion not left on long enough	Re-perm the hair using a weaker perm lotion
Straight pieces of hair	Sections too wide Incorrect angling and placing of perm rods Carelessly leaving out pieces of hair Neutraliser applied unevenly	Re-perm straight pieces of hair, but clip the rest of the hair well away from the perm lotion
Hair too curly	Perm rods used were too small	May be gently relaxed by a senior stylist
Over-processed hair (looks frizzy when wet and straight when dry)	Perm lotion too strong Too much heat used during processing Too much tension used Rods too small	Suggest a course of conditioning treatments and regular haircuts Do not re-perm the hair: it will break off
'Fishhooks' or buckled ends	Poor winding; ends not smoothly wound around the perm rod	These must be cut off
Scalp/skin damage or irritation	Perm lotion or relaxers coming into contact with scalp/skin – if it enters the hair follicle 'pull burns' occur Barrier cream not applied to sensitive skin areas Cuts and abrasions to the scalp	Remove any excess perm lotion or relaxers with water. Apply a soothing moisturising cream to the area
Hair breakage	Too much tension during winding Rubber too tight or twisted Perm lotion or relaxing product too strong Hair over-processed	Suggest a course of reconditioning treatments or restructurants

REMEMBER
Always check with your supervisor that you have chosen the proper correction to match the fault beforehand

TEST YOUR KNOWLEDGE

1 Why is it important to wind the hair evenly?

2 Why should you never wind a perm using excess tension?

3 Name the bonds that are broken when perm lotion is applied to the hair.

4 What is a reducing agent and how does it work?

5 Explain how the amino acid cystine changes to cysteine during the chemical process of perming.

6 Which structural ethnic hair type needs a curl rearranger before perming, and why is it needed?

7 Why is perm lotion always applied to dampened hair?

8 Why would you do:

- a nine-section wind

- a brick wind

- a directional wind?

9 What effect would a cold salon have on the processing time?

10 Why is a perm cap used during processing?

11 Describe three considerations when choosing perm lotions.

12 What is important to remember when perming bleached hair?

13 List the causes and corrections of the following perming problems:

- 'fishhooks' or buckled ends

- over-processed hair

- hair breakage

- scalp/skin damage or irritation

- straight pieces of hair.

14 What are your responsibilities to your client under the COSHH Act during perming and relaxing?

15 Why should you check with your supervisor if you are unsure how to correct any mistakes?

16 Describe two differences between Caucasian and African Caribbean hair structure.

17 Describe the effect relaxing has on tight, curly African Caribbean hair.

18 List the three different chemical types of relaxers available and describe their effects.

19 Explain how the amino acid cystine is affected during relaxing.

20 Why are some relaxers incompatible with others?

21 Why should added heat not be used with hydroxide-based products?

22 List the causes and corrections of the following relaxing problems:

- scalp/skin damage or irritation

- deterioration of hair condition.

Neutralising after perming

Neutralising **permanent waves** is the chemical process of fixing the new curl in the hair. It is a very important process. If it is not done properly then the curl will 'drop', the perm will relax and the hair will become straighter.

Once the 'S'-shaped movement has been formed in the hair, the processing is complete and the hair should be neutralised.

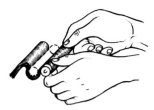

'S' shape to curler size

TO DO

Watch an experienced person in your salon neutralising a perm and make notes on the procedure.

The chemical process of neutralising

The neutralising process is sometimes called **normalising** (returning the hair back to normal) and sometimes called oxidising (because oxygen is added during the process).

The chemical process of neutralising is an oxidation process – all neutralisers contain oxygen. The active ingredient in the neutraliser, which gives off the oxygen, is a weak solution of **hydrogen peroxide** or **sodium bromate**.

The oxygen combines with the hydrogen (which has been released from the reducing agent in perm lotion) to form water. This is why the hair takes longer to dry after a perm: it contains so much water.

The disulphide bonds rejoin in their new permed shape. At the same time the two cysteine molecules become cystine molecules again.

Evidence of really poor neutralising will be instantly recognisable when the hair is ready for styling.

Sodium bromate
Sodium bromate is used mainly in acid perm neutralisers because it is less irritating to the skin.

It is most suitable for African Caribbean type hair as it minimises hair discolouration. Due to the strength of the **oxidising agent**, processing time is increased.

Sodium bromate = 5 per cent

Hydrogen peroxide
This is the most commonly used oxidising agent, mainly used in alkaline perms. It works faster than sodium bromate, therefore timing is shorter.

Hydrogen peroxide = 6 per cent or 20 volume

As neutralisers may contain differing oxidation agents, it is very important to make sure the correct neutraliser for the perm is being used.

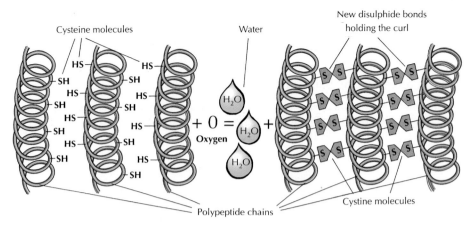

Cysteine molecules

Water

New disulphide bonds holding the curl

HS— SH HS— SH HS— SH HS— SH HS— SH HS— SH

$+ \text{O} = $ Oxygen $+ $

H_2O

H_2O

H_2O

S S S S

Polypeptide chains

Cystine molecules

Neutralising

TO DO

Read the manufacturer's instructions on some neutraliser in your salon and make notes on the ingredients.

Rinsing the hair before applying neutraliser

Take the client to the wash-basin (a back wash-basin is preferable as there is less likelihood of chemicals running into the client's eyes) and make sure the client is both comfortable and correctly gowned for neutralising (sometimes a protective disposable plastic cape is used around the shoulders).

Test the water temperature on the inside of your wrist and check the temperature during rinsing by keeping one of your fingers under the water spray. Ask the client if the temperature is comfortable, then make sure you thoroughly rinse all the curlers on the head. Use your free hand to cup the water over the rods and let it run back down into the wash-basin. Continue rinsing until all the perm solution has been rinsed out of the hair. This will take a minimum of five minutes.

Removing excess water from the wound hair

This is also called 'blotting' the hair and should always be done before the neutraliser is applied. Use either a dry absorbent towel or a wad of cotton wool and press carefully into the rods so as not to disturb them. Remember the hair is still very soft and fragile at this stage.

REMEMBER

Any excess water left in the hair before neutralising will dilute the neutraliser and it will not work properly.

Up to 60 ml of water can be removed during 'blotting', so do it thoroughly.

Water temperature
Water temperature when neutralising should be warm, not hot, to prevent burning and client discomfort and also sudden perm curl tightening.

TO DO

● *Check the manufacturer's instructions on all of the neutralisers in your salon. Make notes on the mixing and timing.*

Mixing the neutraliser

- Always make sure you have the correct neutraliser for the perm that has been used (and that you have not picked up the perm lotion by mistake).
- Some neutralisers have to be measured out or need mixing, so always check the amounts needed; you may need more for long hair.
- Make sure you have the correct equipment with which to apply the neutraliser. Some lotions are foamed up in a large bowl with a neutraliser sponge, some are applied to the hair then foamed up with a sponge on the rods, others are poured directly on to the hair from a bottle with a special applicator nozzle.

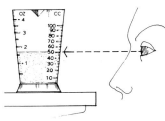

Mixing the neutraliser

Applying the neutraliser

The neutraliser must be thoroughly applied so that every single rod is covered with the solution. You will normally need to use about two-thirds of the amount, saving the last third to use once the rods have been removed from the hair.

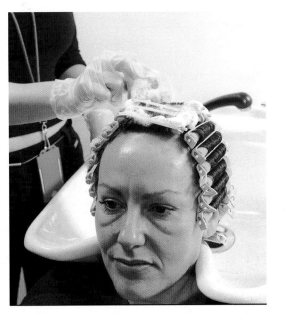

Applying the neutraliser

Timing

Timing is very important, as under-neutralising results in the rebuilding of fewer cystine linkages within the disulphide bonds, therefore the hair curl movement is weak. Over-neutralising changes cystine into cysteric acid, which does not form **cross-linkages**, again weakening the hair structure.

Most neutralisers are left on for about five minutes. The timing is very important. If you are not sure, either check the manufacturer's instructions again or ask your supervisor. If the neutraliser is not left on long enough, the disulphide bonds will not have time to reform and the hair will go straight.

Unwinding the curlers

When the oxidation is complete (after five minutes), each rod should be gently removed without applying any tension or pulling the hair. Always start removing the rods from underneath, at the nape area, and work carefully, removing one rod at a time.

You can now apply the remaining neutraliser (one-third of the original amount) to the ends of the hair. To make sure that all the hair has absorbed the neutraliser solution, leave it on for a few more minutes or longer for long hair while you rinse and dry the perm rods and dispose of the end papers.

Rinsing the hair after neutralising

Test the temperature of the water – remember that the client's scalp may be a little tender, so do not have the water too hot.

Rinse the hair thoroughly and apply a post-perm, anti-oxidant conditioner to prevent creeping oxidation and prevent it from becoming dehydrated.

TO DO

- Check the manufacturer's instructions of all the post-perm conditioners in your salon.
- Make notes on their applications and timing.

An acid-balanced conditioner is helpful after perming to return the hair to its normal pH-balanced, acid state.

Effect on colour

Sometimes neutralisers have the effect of lightening or fading hair colour. This happens particularly if the hair is porous or has been permanently coloured (tinted). The easiest remedy is to use a matching temporary or semi-permanent colour, but check with your supervisor which colour would be best.

Neutralising shampoos for relaxers

The hair must be shampooed thoroughly with neutralising shampoo to remove excess relaxer from the hair and scalp and to stop the action of the relaxer.

On the second shampoo, comb the hair straight, using gentle pressure to prevent damage to the scalp and gentle tension to prevent excessive pulling on the softened hair length.

Leave for five minutes, then rinse thoroughly.

Always check for understanding of the manufacturer's instructions regarding neutralising methods; some products change colour to show that the neutralising is complete.

Blot the hair, then use a pH-balanced moisturising conditioner as a post-relaxing treatment, leave for 10 minutes, then rinse thoroughly.

TO DO

Read the section in Chapter 3 on the disposal of waste materials.

REMEMBER

The hair is still in a softened state, so never pull the rods out of the hair. Always work gently or you will straighten the perm.

REMEMBER

Neutralising shampoos work differently from perm neutralisers.

Never use a neutralising shampoo after a normal perm as it doesn't contain any oxygen to fix the new curl in shape. Similarly, never use a a perm neutraliser after relaxing as this would add extra, unnecessary oxygen to the hair.

1   Give two other names for the chemical process of neutralising.

2   What does the oxygen from the neutraliser form in the hair during the 'fixing stage'?

3   What happens to the cysteine molecules during neutralising?

4   What are your responsibilities under the 1992 COSHH Regulations during neutralising?

5   Why is it important to time both the rinsing (the removal of perm lotion) and the neutraliser product?

6   Why is it important to unwind the perm rods gently?

7   Name the two chemical ingredients often found in neutralisers.

8   What can happen to the hair colour during neutralising?

9   What would happen if you used a neutralising shampoo instead of a neutraliser after perming?

10 List the causes of scalp or skin damage or irritation and how they can be corrected.

11 What is the effect of using a neutralising shampoo on hair that has just been relaxed?

12 Why is it important that neutralising shampoos, not perming neutralisers, are used after relaxing?

13 Why is it important to time the neutralising shampoo?

14 Why must the hair be combed straight on the second neutralising shampoo?

15 How and why should waste materials be disposed of correctly?

16 Why is it important to test the temperature of the water before neutralising?

17 What effect does a post-perm, pH-balanced conditioner have on the hair?

Record cards

TO DO

Re-read the section in Chapter 1 on the Data Protection Act, then ask your supervisor if you have completed your records correctly.

The perming record card is normally completed after perming but before styling and should then be filed away.

REMEMBER

Always check the name *and address* of the client: you may have 10 clients called 'Mrs Brown'.

Permanent waving record card

Client name:

Address:

Daytime tel. no.:

Date of 1st perm: _____

Colour treated or natural: _____

If treated, product: _____

Texture: _____

Condition: _____

Date	Type of lotion	Lotion strength	Size of curlers	Result required	Development time and method	Special notes	Neutralising time and method	Conditioner	Result obtained	Stylist

Perming record card

Relaxer Record Card

Client name
_____
_____

Address
_____
_____
_____

Daytime telephone number
_____
_____

Date of 1st relaxer	**Date**	**Special notes**
Colour treated/natural	**Make of relaxer**	
If treated, product used	**Product strength**	**Neutralising time and method**
Texture	**Virgin head or regrowth**	**Conditioner**
Condition	**Result required**	**Result obtained**
	Development time and method	**Stylist**

Relaxer record card

Chapter 10 Colouring and bleaching

After working through this chapter you will be able to:

- Understand the basic techniques for colouring
- Carry out appropriate tests
- Add colour and permanently change hair colour using the correct products, tools and equipment
- Understand how skin tone, hair condition and style can affect the overall result.

This chapter covers the following NVQ Level 2 unit:
Change Hair Colour Using Basic Techniques

Introduction

Colouring and bleaching hair are a very exciting part of hairdressing. You can change the client's hair colour quite subtly just by covering a few **grey hairs**, or very dramatically by turning a mousy brown into a glamorous **blonde**!

Many hairdressers are frightened of applying colour because they do not understand the theory behind it. Here are just two examples.

- You cannot put a light ash blonde tint on a dark brown head of hair and expect it to come out blonde. You need to bleach it first.
- You cannot put a rich auburn colour on a client with a head of naturally white hair; their hair will turn out a very bright red. You need to mix in some brown with the rich auburn colour.

DURATION	TYPE OF COLOURANT
One wash	Temporary colours, e.g. coloured mousse and coloured setting lotions. These are used to enhance the present hair colour.
6–8 washes	Semi-permanent colours – these colour and condition the hair and gradually fade away. They are not mixed with hydrogen peroxide.
15–20 washes	**Quasi-permanent** colours – these are stronger than semi-permanent colours. They give a better coverage of white hair and a good shine. They are mixed with developers (which are a low strength of hydrogen peroxide) and do leave a slight regrowth. These need a skin test.
Grow out of the hair	Permanent colours, i.e. tints. These have the best and broadest range of colours, can lighten, darken and give lots of different **tones** and leave the hair in very good condition. They can be used for both full-head colours and **lowlights**. High-lift tints, which lighten the hair more than normal tints, but not as much as bleach, are often used for highlighting. These need a skin test. Bleaches – these remove colour from the hair, especially from dark hair when high-lift tints are not strong enough. Bleaches can be used both for full-head lightening and for highlights.

TO DO

Find the colour charts in your salon and ask your supervisor which ones are:
* *temporary colours*
* *semi-permanent colours*
* *permanent colours*
* *products used to lighten hair.*
Make a note of each for future use.

Establishing hair colour

Lighting

Light plays a very important part in the appearance of hair colours. If you are sitting in a darkened room such as a cinema, then you cannot see the true colour of the hair of the person next to you until the lights come on. In the same way you cannot see the true colour of your client's hair if you do not have good lighting in your salon.

The best light in which to look at hair colour is natural daylight. If your salon has lots of large windows and white walls, then you should be able to see hair colour quite well.

However, if the salon has lots of dark walls or poor lighting, then you may have to take the client over to a window or show them the true colour (especially coppers and reds) with a hand mirror.

Natural hair colour

There are two types of natural hair colour.

White hair

This contains no colour pigments at all. Remember, there is no such thing as grey hair – it is white hair mixed with naturally coloured hair. For example, light brown

HEALTH MATTERS

Assessing the client's hair colour is a critical part of hair colouring, so try to organise your workstation without glare so that you are not looking directly into the light, at a white wall or a mirror reflecting either. Glare can be both irritating and tiring to your eyes.

hair and white hair looks salt and pepper colour, dark brown hair and white hair looks steel grey.

Naturally coloured hair

This contains colour pigments found in the cortex. It is known as 'virgin hair', which means that it has never been artificially coloured.

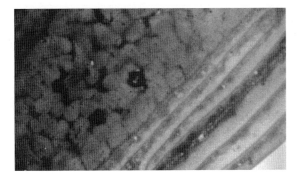

Colour pigments in the cortex

Hair pigment

The two main types of pigment found in hair are:

- melanin (sometimes called granular pigment), which is brown or black
- pheomelanin (sometimes called diffuse pigment), which is red or yellow.

The amount of melanin and pheomelanin present in hair depends upon the hair colour

Natural hair colour	Pigment mixture
Black	Mostly black
Dark brown	Red, brown, black
Light brown	Yellow, red, brown
Blonde	Yellow, red
White	No pigment

The colour pigment melanin is formed in the melanocytes by the oxidation of the amino acid tyrosine. Tyrosine is a mixture of protein and copper.

Lack of hair colour can be caused by the following:

- lack of protein in the body
- lack of copper in the body
- the body's inability to produce tyrasinase, due to old age.

The condition albinism is the body's genetic failure to manufacture tyrosine.

To change the colour of hair, new pigments are added: sometimes to the surface of the hair (temporary and semi-permanent colours); and sometimes to the hair cortex (permanent colours).

To lighten the natural hair colour the pigments are bleached out.

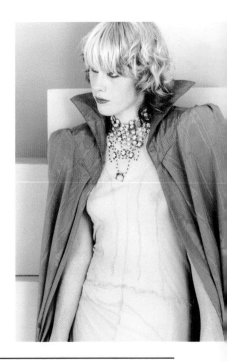

Hair texture and porosity related to hair colour

Hair that is more porous because it has been permed, relaxed or highlighted, or that is in a generally damaged condition, will absorb colour more quickly in some areas – giving an **uneven colour** as a result. Remember also that colours will fade more quickly on porous hair.

Very coarse-textured hair (such as strong white hair) can be resistant to colour, so you may need to do a test cutting.

TO DO

Re-read the section in Chapter 1 on porosity tests, elasticity tests, test cuttings, incompatability tests, strand tests and skin tests. Make brief notes on how to do each one and summarise the purpose of each.

Choosing the right colour

Skin tones

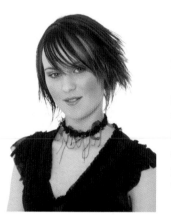

Skin tones are either warm with peachy yellow undertones or cool with pink undertones. Eye colour can give a good indication of a warm or cool skin tone – blue or grey eyes for **cool tones** and brown/hazel or green eyes for **warm tones**. Although we keep our skin tones for life, unchanged by tanning or age, younger people can take most colours, but as we get older and fine lines and wrinkles appear we need softer colours to complement our skin.

TO DO

- *Find a cool, pink-coloured piece of fabric and a warm, peach-coloured piece of fabric. Working in pairs, drape each piece of material around your partner's neck and look at their face. Look at the whites of the eyes, the shadowing around the mouth and eyes, the appearance of blemishes, lines and wrinkles. The right tone should make the whites of the eyes and skin look clearer, lines, blemishes and wrinkles disappear and there will be a general lifting of the face.*
- *Dark or ashen colours can be very ageing on older clients. They may wish to return their hair to its natural colour in order to look younger, but this is not usually successful as the colour they had then may not always suit them in the present.*

Shade and depth of colour

You will have to learn to train your eye to look at hair colours for two things.

- The **depth** of colour. This is how light or how dark the hair is – very light blonde, blonde, light brown, medium brown, etc. This is also called the **base shade**.
- The tone of colour. This is the shade of colour on a particular depth – light ash blonde, light golden blonde, light warm blonde, light silver blonde.

- *Using your salon's permanent colour chart, try to match the colours of your clients' hair to the colours shown on the chart.*
- *Make a note of each colour number on the chart and its corresponding description.*

The International Colour Chart System (ICC)

Most manufacturers use a numbering system called the 'International Colour Chart System' for choosing colours. This is so that hairdressers can be precise when choosing colours. For example, your idea of red may be a rich auburn colour, but your client's idea of red may be a pale copper colour, so you will need to use a colour chart to achieve exactly the colour your client wants.

◄───── Tone (shades of the basic colour) ─────►

Tone / Depth	.1 (Blue) Ash	.2 (Violet) Mauve Ash	.3 (Yellow) Golden	.4 (Orange) Copper	.5 (Red) Mahogany	.6 (Red) Red
10 Lightest blonde						
9 Very light blonde	e.g. very light ash blonde 9.1					
8 Light blonde						
7 Blonde			e.g. golden blonde 7.3			
6 Dark blonde						
5 Light brown				e.g. light copper brown 5.4		
4 Brown						
3 Dark brown						
2 Very dark brown						
1 Black						

(left axis label: Depth (base colours))

Example of an ICC colour chart

Above is an example of an ICC chart. You can see that the depth of colours (or base colours) are numbered from 1 to 10 and the tones of colours are numbered as .1, .2, .3, .4, .5, .6. Some examples are already written in – e.g. 9.1 is a very light ash blonde, because 9 is a very light blonde and .1 is ash.

Using the chart above, work out what colours 7.2, 4.4 and 10.1 would be.

Extra information

Some colours have two numbers after the depth, e.g. 8.31, 9.33, 6.01.

- The first number after the point is the strongest tone, e.g. 8.31 is light golden blonde (the 8 and the 3), with a little ash tone (the 1).
- If the second number after the point is the same number as the first, then the tone is twice as concentrated (twice as bright), e.g. 9.33.
- If the first number after the point is a 0, e.g. 6.01, then the tone is diluted, e.g. dark natural ash blonde.

Not all manufacturers list their colour tones as numbers: some have letters such as G for Gold, R for Red.

As a professional hair colourist you should become familiar with at least one product range to enable you to be able to intermix the colours from that particular range, hence giving you a wider choice of colours.

TO DO

- *Try to learn all the names of the colour depths and their numbers on your salon's colour chart.*
- *Make yourself familiar with all of the colour tones on your salon's colour chart.*

Summary of points to remember when choosing a hair colour

Client's requirements

- How light or dark (depth) do they want the colour?
- What tone do they want, e.g. red, copper, ashen?
- Use the shade chart to decide together with the client.

Client's natural (base) colour

Very dark hair cannot be tinted to light blonde (you will have to pre-lighten with bleach).

Amount of white hair present

The more white hair the brighter any warm tones such as red and copper will show up.

Hair condition and porosity

Unevenly porous hair will absorb colours unevenly.

Hair texture and density

Some coarse-textured hair is resistant to colouring (take a test cutting first).

In the chemical process of hair colouring the cuticle scales swell, adding more texture to the hair, making it ideal for giving more manageability to fine, resistant hair. Varying the amount of colour, high- or lowlights in the hair, can control this texture. The more high- or lowlights added to the hair, the more volume and texture the hair will have.

Complexion and skin tones

Never colour an older client's hair too dark or too ash – it will make them look older.

African Caribbean hair

Natural African Caribbean hair is not as fragile as chemically treated hair, so any colouring processes should be similar to European hair colouring.

Care must be taken if the hair has previously been chemically treated, e.g. relaxed, as this will require extra careful attention if colouring is to take place.

Time and money

Make sure the client knows how much time is involved – for example, foil highlights can take $1\frac{1}{2}$ hours plus drying time. Ask the client if they are aware of the prices of various colour services; if not show them the price list. If the client has long or thick hair and more product is needed, ask your supervisor to quote a price before you start.

The colour spectrum

Light from the sun is made up of a mixture of colours, which can be seen naturally in a rainbow. These colours – red, orange, yellow, green, blue, indigo and violet – make up the colour spectrum.

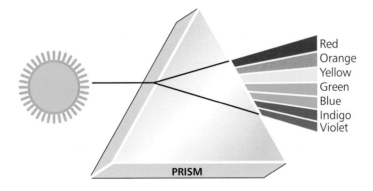

Light split into the spectrum

You can see all these colours easily when you look through a cut-glass prism. There is a mnemonic to remember the colours: 'Richard Of York Gave Battle In Vain'.

These same colours are used as colour pigments in hair colouring. The **colour star** shows how they are related to the colour tones that hairdressers use.

For example, you would not say to a client, 'I'm going to put orange on your hair'; you would say, 'I'm going to put a copper tone on your hair'.

You have to know about these tones because the colours opposite each other on the star cancel each other out. If a client's hair becomes too red, you apply green (matt); if a client's hair becomes too orange, you apply blue (ash); if it becomes too yellow (this may happen after highlights), you apply violet (silver).

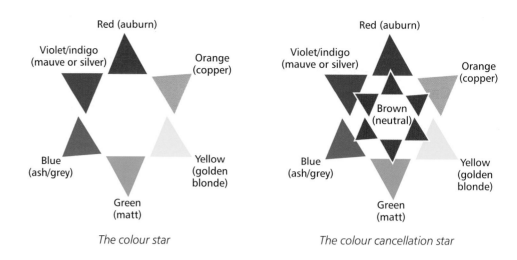

REMEMBER

When cancelling out colours, the two colours must be the same depth, e.g. pale yellow 9.3 must be masked by 9.2 pale silver to produce pale brown (beige).

REMEMBER

Yellow discolouration is masked by purple (mauve or silver). Orange discolouration is masked by blue (ash). Red discolouration is masked by green (matt).

The colour star

The colour cancellation star

It is not advisable to intermix certain colours as unwanted tones can result, e.g. mixing an ash shade and a copper shade would have a neutralised tone effect.

TO DO

Watch some children washing out their paintbrushes after an art class. All the bright reds, blues, yellows, greens, oranges and mauves will mix together (colour cancellation) to form a sludgy brown or neutral colour.

Using hydrogen peroxide for colouring and bleaching

Hydrogen peroxide is mixed with both permanent colours and hair bleaches. If it were used by itself it would lighten hair colour and make the hair more porous. It is occasionally used to soften very coarse-textured hair before applying a permanent tint.

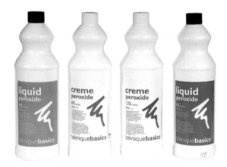

Hydrogen peroxide

TO DO

Read the section in Chapter 3 on the COSHH Act and list all the precautions needed when using hydrogen peroxide, bleaches and colour in the salon.

Once it is mixed with permanent colours or hair bleaches, hydrogen peroxide releases oxygen – it is therefore known as an oxidising agent. The chemical formula for hydrogen peroxide is H_2O_2, and here you can see how it breaks down during mixing:

$$H_2O_2 \qquad \xrightarrow{\text{breaks down to form}} \qquad H_2O + O$$

Hydrogen peroxide   breaks down to form   Water and oxygen

Dilutions of hydrogen peroxide

The following formulae can be used to calculate volume strengths and percentage strengths.

$$\frac{\text{Volume strength}}{10} \times 3 = \text{percentage strength}$$

$$\frac{\text{Percentage strength}}{3} \times 10 = \text{volume strength}$$

Hydrogen peroxide can be purchased at various strengths. The higher the strength the larger the amount of available oxygen, e.g. 1 litre of 30 volume hydrogen peroxide allows 30 litres of oxygen to be released.

Volume strength

Hydrogen peroxide is available in either volume strengths or percentage (%) strengths.

Hydrogen peroxide: strengths and uses

VOLUME STRENGTH (VOL)	PERCENTAGE STRENGTH (%)	USE
10 vol	3%	For adding weak colour (e.g. bleach toners)
20 vol	6%	For adding colour (e.g. for most tinting purposes
30 vol	9%	For lightening hair colour
40 vol	12%	For highlights and highlifting tints
60 vol	18%	For highlights and highlifting tints

Using high volume/percentage strengths on the hair can cause burns and hair breakage.

It may be supplied as either a liquid or a cream, but the strengths are the same.

- Cream peroxides contain thickeners and acid **stabiliser**. The thickeners make the hydrogen peroxide easier to control and use, hence making it less likely to bleed when weaving highlights. The cream consistency helps keep the product moist for longer on the hair.

- Liquid peroxide is a clear, water-like substance with acid stabiliser added to help minimise oxidation until it is mixed with an alkali (tint or bleach), which then speeds up the release of oxygen, leaving water as the residue.

Hydrogen peroxide will not work if it has 'gone off', which means it has lost its strength (and its oxygen). This will happen if it is not stored properly. Therefore you must always:

- keep the containers tightly closed and put the lids back on as soon as possible after use

- measure out the amount of peroxide you need. If you have any left over, do not pour it back into the bottle as it may have picked up some dust
- store it in a cool, dark place.

All peroxides have an acid stabiliser added to them which helps to prevent loss of strength.

REMEMBER

When measuring liquids:
1 fl oz = approx 30 ml.

Sometimes you might have to dilute liquid hydrogen peroxide from a stronger solution to a weaker one. The table below shows the different dilutions.

Dilution of hydrogen peroxide

VOLUME OF HYDROGEN PEROXIDE	PARTS OF HYDROGEN PEROXIDE		PARTS OF DISTILLED WATER	VOLUME PRODUCED
60	2	+	1	40
60	1	+	1	30
60	1	+	2	20
60	1	+	5	10
40	3	+	1	30
40	1	+	1	20
40	1	+	3	10
30	2	+	1	20
30	1	+	2	10
20	1	+	1	10

Preparing the client

Gowning up

It is best to gown up the client with a plastic or rubberised bleaching or tint gown to prevent any chemical splashes reaching the client's clothes. Most salons also use towels, shoulder capes and tissues around the neck area.

When you are using very dark colours or have clients with sensitive skin you may also need to use protective barrier cream around the hairline.

TO DO
- *Re-read the section in Chapter 1 on gowning up and watch someone do this.*
- *Make a note of exactly how to gown up for a colour or bleach in your salon.*

For partial head block colouring, section off the hair that is not being coloured and secure it firmly with section clips. Cover the hair that is not to be coloured with strips of cotton wool, either clipped to the hair or attached to a thin film of barrier cream near the roots.

REMEMBER

Protect your own clothes with a dye apron and wear protective gloves.

Checking the scalp

Always check the client's scalp for any inflammation, cuts or abrasions. If you are in doubt whether to proceed, call your supervisor and tactfully (remembering the client's feelings) ask for advice.

TO DO

Read page 46, which describes the preparation of equipment, to check that you have not forgotten anything. For ease of use, keep your trolley on your right side if you are right-handed (left side if you are left-handed), and avoid any obstruction.

Skin test

Make sure your client has had a skin test if para dyes are to be used (see Chapter 1).

Hair texture and porosity

Check the hair texture and porosity. Remember that some coarse-textured hair can be resistant to colour and unevenly porous hair (dry ends) can absorb colour unevenly. Take a test cutting if you are unsure about the result.

TO DO

- *Read the section in Chapter 3 on the sterilisation of tools and equipment.*
- *List and describe four methods of each.*

Keeping your work area tidy and clean

Not only should you protect yourself and your client from accidental colour and bleach spillages, but you should also check that your surrounding area (which includes the dressing tables, chairs, trollies, equipment, floor and shampoo basins) is kept clean and tidy. Many a smart new outfit has been ruined by a casual brush against product spillages!

Skin and eye damage is another risk to consider, so always work carefully, mopping up any product that falls.

TO DO

Find out your salon's procedures for reporting shortages.

TEST YOUR KNOWLEDGE

1 Why should you prepare and position your tools and equipment properly before starting to colour or bleach hair?

2 Why is it important to keep your work area tidy and clean?

3 Why is it important to report both product stock and sundry shortages to the relevant person?

4 Describe the principles of colouring hair.

5 Describe the principles of colour selection.

Record cards

There is quite a lot of information needed when colouring and bleaching a client's hair, so always complete the record card straight away in case you forget any of the details.

Hair colour record card											
Client name: _____ Natural hair colour: _____											
Address: _____ Texture: _____											
_____ Condition: _____											
Daytime tel. no.: _____											
Skin test: Date: Name of operator:											

RECORD OF APPLICATION

Date	Type	Colour	Hydrogen peroxide	Development		Application special notes	After treatment	Result		Stylist
				Method	Time			Required	Obtained	

Colour record card

TO DO

Re-read the section in Chapter 1 on the Data Protection Act. Complete a colour record card, then ask your supervisor if you have completed your record card correctly.

Temporary colours

Temporary colours are very popular because they create an instant colour change. They are quick to apply and easy to remove if the client is dissatisfied with the result.

Temporary colours are useful for adding stronger tones to natural or artificially coloured light or dark hair, e.g. warm golden, ashen, rich auburn.

Sometimes natural white hair or bleached hair looks too yellow or golden (brassy) and benefits from being neutralised by silver tones.

However, blending in a few grey hairs (remember grey hair is white and naturally coloured hair mixed together) may be more difficult. Some colours produce unwanted warm (orange/red) overtones on white hair.

Temporary colours can also be used to darken natural and artificially coloured hair.

REMEMBER

Temporary colours wash out of the hair the first time you shampoo.

TO DO

- *Use your temporary colour shade chart to match and select several different colours for different clients.*
- *Check your choice with your supervisor. If you are a little unsure either take a test cutting (see Chapter 1) or try out a little of the colour on the underneath of the hair.*
- *Make a note of the colour used on a record card.*

Forms of temporary colours available and their application

COLOURED MOUSSE	COLOURED SETTING LOTION	COLOUR SHAMPOOS	HAIR MASCARAS	COLOURED HAIRSPRAY
Apply to towel-dried hair: shake the container thoroughly, squeeze the nozzle, then apply to the palm of your (gloved) hand and spread over the hair with your fingertips	Apply to towel-dried hair: either sprinkle on the hair from the bottle or (to even out colour on more porous hair) apply to small sections with a bowl and brush. These lotions also help to keep the set in place	These are shampooed on to the hair at the basin to enhance the hair colour. They are rinsed out and do not contain styling aids	Applied on to dry hair after styling with a brush similar to, but larger than, a mascara brush	Spray on to dry hair after styling. Remember to protect other areas (such as the client's face) with tissue when spraying

The chemistry of temporary colours

The pigment molecules of temporary colours (azo dyes) are too large to enter the hair shaft, so they coat the outside of the hair. This is why they are washed away so easily.

However, unevenly porous hair (e.g. permed and highlighted ends) will always take a temporary colour unevenly. The cuticle scales are swollen and open in porous, chemically treated hair and the large colour molecules can become trapped there and do not wash out.

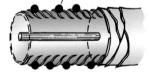

Colour molecule

The chemical action of temporary colours

TEST YOUR KNOWLEDGE

1. What types of temporary colours are available in your salon?
2. What colour tone would you recommend for a client whose blonde highlights are too yellow?
3. Name the part of the hair that is affected by temporary colour.
4. How long should a temporary colour last on the hair?
5. State how the client's natural hair colour depth and tone will affect the temporary colour result, including the percentage of white hair.
6. State the effect of applying a temporary hair colour to unevenly porous, chemically treated hair.

REMEMBER

All temporary colours are quick to apply because they do not need a development time and they do not need to be removed: the process should take no longer than 15 minutes.

Semi-permanent colours

Semi-permanent colours have the advantage of colouring and conditioning hair at the same time. They do not need to be mixed with hydrogen peroxide and so do not leave any regrowth.

They are useful for blending in a small amount of white (grey) hair, but are not strong enough colours to cover a lot of white hair.

TO DO

- *Use your semi-permanent colour shade chart to match and select several different colours for different clients, including very light blonde, medium brown and very dark brown base shades.*
- *Check your choice with your supervisor. If you are a little unsure about the result then take a test cutting (see Chapter 1) and show the result to your client.*

REMEMBER

Semi-permanent colours last 6–8 shampoos and do not leave a regrowth.

The chemistry of semi-permanent colours

The pigment molecules of semi-permanent colours (nitro dyes) are smaller than those of temporary colours and so are able to penetrate a little way into the cortex of the hair. They tend to wash out slowly and so last longer than temporary colours.

Unevenly porous hair (e.g. chemically treated, permed, relaxed or bleached hair) will also take a semi-permanent colour unevenly. The cuticle scales are swollen and open in porous hair and the smaller molecules can penetrate deeper into the cortex in the porous part of the hair, although they rinse off normally from the non-porous parts – producing patchy results.

Preparing the client

- Re-read the section on pages 238–239 on preparing the client for colouring or bleaching. Assess the amount of white hair present. Semi-permanents will cover only a small amount of white hair. Take a test cutting if you are unsure of the result.
- Pay special attention when gowning up for semi-permanent colours because they are stain dyes. They will stain your hands or your client's skin in the same way that a felt-tip pen stains. So make sure you wear gloves and protect your client's skin with barrier cream.

TO DO

Check the manufacturer's instructions on the semi-permanent and quasi-permanent colours in your salon to see if any of them require a skin test to be carried out.

- Check the manufacturer's instructions before shampooing. You normally give one or two shampoos – but no conditioner – then towel dry the hair before applying the product.
- Also check the manufacturer's instructions for mixing. Some products are applied directly from the bottle, tube or flask, while others are poured into a bowl and applied with a sponge or brush.

Application methods

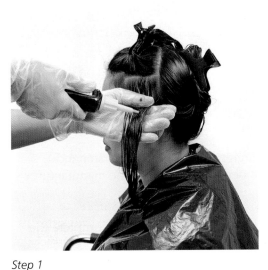

Step 1

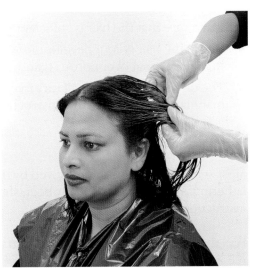

Step 2

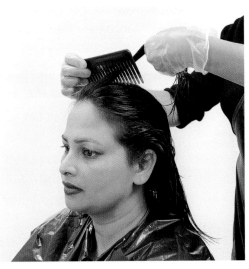

Step 3

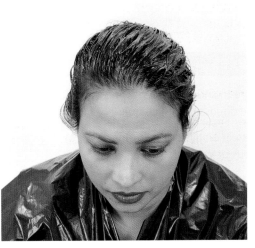

Step 4

- Use the correct amount of product for the length of hair (short hair needs less than long hair). Check with your supervisor if you are in doubt about how much to use.
- Mix or prepare the colour according to the manufacturer's instructions.
- Divide the hair into four large sub-sections and secure with section clips.
- Take neat, even partings for the sub-sections. Hair that is generally thick and products with a thick consistency need smaller sections and vice versa.

- Start working from the crown downwards and keep the hair controlled so that it does not fall on the client's skin.
- Speed is very important when applying semi-permanent colours as they do not take long to process or develop.
- When you have finished, cross-check the application (check by taking sections in the opposite direction from the way in which you applied it). Remove any skin staining with damp cotton wool immediately.

Developing and timing the colour

- Make sure that the hair is sufficiently loosened to allow the circulation of air.
- Check the hair colour development by taking a strand test (see Chapter 1). Remember that over-porous hair develops quickly.
- The development time will vary from five to 45 minutes, depending on the manufacturer, so check the instructions.

Removing the colour

Most semi-permanents are removed by thorough rinsing with warm water and lathering, as the hair has already been shampooed. (Always check the manufacturer's instructions to make sure.)

Feel the hair to make sure it is clean and use a conditioner if needed. Complete the record card.

REMEMBER

Always check with your supervisor that you have chosen the proper correction to match the fault before attempting the correction.

Summary of semi-permanent colour faults and corrections

FAULT	CAUSES	CORRECTION
Incorrect colour result	Failure to show the client the shade chart while discussing the colour	Shampoo repeatedly until the colour has faded
	Incorrect analysis of hair (not noticing strong, porous or white hair)	
	Not taking a test cutting	
	Under- or over-developing semi-permanent colours	
Skin staining	Colour used on a very dry scalp	Remove with dampened cotton wool or skin stain remover
	Barrier cream not used around the client's hairline	
Patchy result	Poor application	Shampoo repeatedly until the colour has faded. If this does not work then try using either white spirit and cotton wool to dry hair or a **brightening shampoo** (equal parts 10 vol peroxide and shampoo), or try a bleach bath (equal parts powder bleach/warm water and shampoo)
	Sections too large	
	Application not checked	
	Unevenly porous hair: has absorbed the colour unevenly and become patchy	

1 Why is gowning up especially important when using semi-permanent colour?

2 State how skin staining is best avoided when applying semi-permanent colours.

3 What is the average length of time that a semi-permanent colour should last?

4 What is the difference between applying a semi-permanent colour and a temporary colour?

5 Which parts of the hair are affected by semi-permanent colours?

6 State how the client's natural hair colour depth and tone will affect the semi-permanent colour result, including the percentage of white hair.

7 State the effect of applying a semi-permanent colour to unevenly porous, chemically treated hair.

8 Describe two correction methods that may be used if the semi-permanent colour has produced uneven results.

9 What are your responsibilities to your client under the COSHH Act?

10 Why should you check with your supervisor if you are unsure about how to correct any mistakes?

Quasi-permanent colours

Quasi-permanent colours are also known as deposit-only colours, tone-on-tone colours or oxy-permanents.

This type of hair colouring lasts longer than a semi-permanent, approximately 15–20 shampoos, but not as long as a permanent tint.

The chemistry of quasi-permanent colours

These types of colours have small and medium-sized pigment molecules; the smaller molecules are able to slightly penetrate the cortex, while the medium-sized molecules penetrate the cuticle.

To become active, quasi-permanents must be mixed with an oxidation agent or developer such as low-volume hydrogen peroxide. The purpose of the developer is to open the cuticle layer and allow the smaller colour molecules to penetrate to the cortex.

This gives the kindness of a semi-permanent with the durability of a permanent; they do leave a slight regrowth.

Due to the low oxidation strength of the developer, 1–3%, these are non-lightening colours, only capable of darkening or adding tone to natural hair, making it ideal for translucent covering of white hair, corrective colouring and lowlighting, and to refresh permanent tints.

It is important to remember that colour on top of colour will always appear darker. Therefore if a tone only change is needed, choose a shade one level lighter than the client's colour.

Hair porosity must always be taken into account when applying quasi-permanents as porous hair could produce patchy results.

Mixing ratio is usually 1:2 (1 part product:2 parts developer), using the developer designed for the product.

The procedure to follow is the same as for a semi-permanent application (see pages 243–244). Always follow the manufacturer's instructions regarding mixing, application and timing guidelines.

Permanent colours

There are three main types of permanent hair colour.

Natural vegetable dyes

The most common of these is **henna** (Lawsone), which gives copper or red tones to the hair. It works by coating the hair shaft and sticking to the outside cuticle layer. Brown and black henna colours are created when metallic sorts are mixed with the henna; this mixture is known as compound henna or compound colours.

Clients often use henna at home because it shows up well on dark hair and gives body and shine. If a client has had many applications of henna, then a build-up occurs. This can be a problem if perms, relaxers or permanent colours are requested, as they cannot penetrate through the henna coating to work inside the cortex. If in doubt, take a test cutting first.

Metallic dyes

These are sold in shops as hair colour restorers (e.g. Grecian 2000). Never perm, tint or bleach over hair dyed with metallic dyes – it will break off. (Re-read the section in Chapter 1 on incompatibility tests.)

Synthetic dyes

Permanent tints are para dyes and are known as oxidation dyes because they are always mixed with hydrogen peroxide.

The widest possible choice of colours is available with permanent tints. They can be used to darken or lighten (up to four shades lighter), and have a whole range of subtle and vibrant tones (see the ICC chart on page 233).

TO DO

- Use your permanent colour shade chart to match and select several different colours for different clients.
- Check your choice with your supervisor.
- If you are not quite sure about the result, take a test cutting (see Chapter 1) and show the result to your client.

Forms of tint available

Creams (tube)

These are mixed to a creamy consistency and are particularly good for covering coarse, resistant hair.

Oil-based tints (bottle)

These liquids mix to a gel-like thickness and give a more natural, finished look.

Oil/cream emulsion (tube/bottle)

These have the benefits of both creams and gel tints and are easy to work with.

Mixing tints

All tints are mixed with hydrogen peroxide (either liquid or cream) and often in equal parts, e.g. 60 ml of tint and 60 ml of hydrogen peroxide.

Mix your tint just a few minutes before you need to use it – it will 'go off' if you mix it too soon.

TO DO

Look up the section on hydrogen peroxide on page 236 of this chapter to check the different uses for different strengths of peroxide (e.g. 10, 20, 30, 40 and 60 vol).

The chemistry of permanent tints

Tints are alkaline so will swell the hair and open up the cuticle scales, allowing the colour to enter the cortex.

All tints are made of small molecules of para dye mixed with hydrogen peroxide. These small molecules of tint link with the hydrogen peroxide inside the hair shaft to form larger molecules that cannot escape. This is called an oxidation reaction.

Once the colour has developed it remains permanently inside the hair shaft, and an acid anti-oxy rinse is applied after shampooing to close down the cuticle scales.

REMEMBER

Permanent colours last until they grow out. Regrowth tints need to be reapplied every 4–6 weeks.

REMEMBER

Always check the manufacturer's instructions for the amount of peroxide to add to the tint.

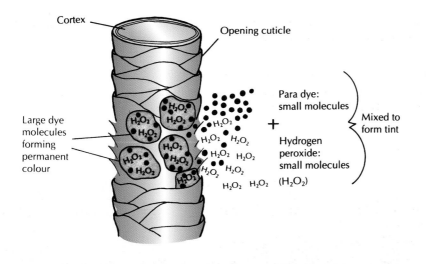

The chemistry of permanent colours

TO DO

Read the labels on the containers of permanent tints in your salon to see the ingredients and whether they contain the word para.

Preparing the client

- Re-read the section on preparing the client for colouring and bleaching (pages 238–239).

- Assess the amount of white hair present – remember, bright colours will show up stronger on white hair. Again, if you are unsure, either check with your supervisor or take a test cutting.

- Do not shampoo before a tint unless the hair is excessively greasy or full of hairspray, in which case you should shampoo and dry the hair thoroughly. The only other exception is when you are going to apply bleach toners to towel-dried hair.

- Use the correct amount of tint. Half a tube is usually sufficient for a regrowth while a whole tube should normally be used for a (short) whole-head, very thick hair or comb-through application.

- Wear gloves to prevent dermatitis.

Application methods

Always divide the hair into equal sections (usually four).

Regrowth application

Take neat, even partings for the sub-sections. Thick hair and products with a thick consistency need smaller sections, and vice versa.

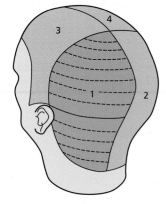

Hair division

Apply the tint to the roots, starting at the back using 6 mm partings. However, if there is any resistant white hair at the front you should start in that area. Do not overlap with the previously tinted hair or the colour will be uneven and patchy. You need to work in a neat, speedy manner without spilling or splashing the tint.

TO DO

Practise applying a thick conditioning cream to a model's hair at the roots only and time yourself. It should not take more than 20 minutes.

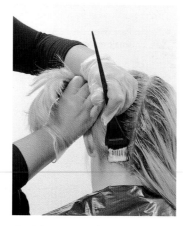

Applying regrowth tint – vertically

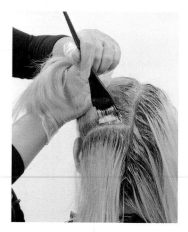

Applying regrowth tint – horizontally

Check the application by sectioning in the opposite direction and reapplying to any uncovered areas.

If the ends are faded the colour may need to be combed through. This is not done every time as it damages the hair, making it more porous. Normally, diluted tint is applied to the ends for the last few minutes of the development time, and the hair massaged with the fingers to distribute the tint evenly.

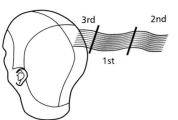

Whole-head application

Whole-head application

For a whole-head application the tint is always applied to the mid-lengths and ends, then to the roots of the hair unless the hair is very short. This is because heat from the client's scalp will make the tint take more quickly on the roots and speeds up the processing time.

Developing and timing the tint

- Make sure that the hair is sufficiently loosened to allow the circulation of air.
- Check the manufacturer's instructions to see how long it should be left before checking (the average time is 30 minutes), and whether you should use heat (from an accelerator), which will halve the development time.
- Check the colour development by taking a strand test (see Chapter 1). Remove some of the colour from the roots and the ends and compare the two colours. If they are of the required shade then remove the colour.

Removing the tint

Take the client to the wash-basin and add a small amount of water to **emulsify** and loosen the colour, while massaging the product, paying attention to the hairline as damp tint will help lift off skin staining when massaged at this time.

The massage movements help mix colouring products with water to form an emulsion, making it easier to remove from the hair.

Rinse off the tint thoroughly with tepid water until the water runs clear. Use a cream or an acid-balanced shampoo, massage gently, then rinse. Apply a second shampoo if necessary.

Use of conditioners

Leave-in conditioners or porosity balancers can be applied to help even out porous hair when applying to temporary and semi-permanent colours.

Use an acid anti-oxy conditioning rinse to prevent the tint from oxidising any further and to close the cuticle scales. To finish, complete the client's record card.

Colour after-care advice

Recommend a specialist shampoo and/or conditioner for the client's hair type and condition.

Advise when the colour process should be repeated.

Give advice on styling tools and equipment such as dryers, brushes, combs and thermally heated tools such as tongs.

Explain the adverse effects of such things on the hair as chlorine, salt water, sun and wind. Advise on protecting the hair when sunbathing and rinsing thoroughly after swimming.

REMEMBER

A warm salon will make the tint take quicker; a cold salon will make the tint take more slowly. Use any waiting time to clear up and write up your record card.

REMEMBER

Always check with your supervisor that you have chosen the proper correction to match the fault before you attempt the correction.

FAULT	CAUSES	CORRECTION
Colour too light	Tint not left on long enough: under-processed Hydrogen peroxide too weak: colour molecules not developed properly Hydrogen peroxide too strong for the amount of tint required	Re-tint the hair using the correct strength of peroxide and developing for the correct length of time
Insufficient coverage	Strong coarse hair (often white) Peroxide strength weakened during process Make-up or barrier cream on the hairline	**Pre-soften** with 10 vol peroxide then apply tint and peroxide mixed Re-apply with fresh tint and peroxide Clean with spirit and reapply tint
Colour too dark	Colour choice too dark Over-porous hair (perhaps from too many comb-throughs)	The hair can be lightened with either a colour reducer or a softening shampoo (a mix of 1 scoop powder bleach/30 ml 6% or 9% peroxide/60 ml warm water/15 ml shampoo), but this must be done by a senior member of staff
Patchy, uneven colour	Uneven application, overlapping, sections too large, insufficient tint used No allowance for body heat on a whole-head application Tint mixed badly, lumps left in the mixture Application too slow Unevenly porous hair	Correct by spot tinting to the lighter areas
Scalp irritated	Peroxide too strong Allergic reaction to tint	Immediately remove with cool water
Colour too ash (green)	Not pre-pigmenting (i.e. using a warm colour before applying the base shade when returning a bleached/lightened client to their natural colour) Chlorine from swimming pools	Bleach bath (a mix of equal parts powder bleach/warm water/shampoo) to cleanse and remove the ash tone
Colour too red	Colour choice too red Too much white hair present Natural warmth in the hair	Re-tint with a matt (green) colour of the same depth
Colour too orange	Colour choice too orange (copper) Too much white hair present Natural warmth in the hair	Re-tint with an ash (blue) colour of the same depth
Colour too yellow	Colour choice too golden Too much white hair present Natural warmth in the hair Peroxide too strong	Re-tint with a silver (violet) colour of the same depth

Bleaching hair

Hairdressers use bleach to lighten hair when other products such as highlifting tints are not strong enough.

Clients who have naturally 'mousy' hair that lightens in the sunlight may wish to achieve this effect by bleaching. Blonde hair is often considered to be more flattering, especially with sun-tanned skin, and once clients have experienced being blonde they often feel that their own colour is less exciting.

Blonde highlights, especially on layered hair (where the natural coloured regrowth is less obvious), are easier to sell to clients. The initial cost of highlights, especially woven highlights (which take more time) may be high, but they need to be repeated only every few months. If clients prefer a full head bleach, then the regrowth must be done every few weeks.

REMEMBER

Bleaching is a permanent process. It will not wash out of the hair.

Bleaching products

Temporary lighteners

To lighten the hair means to remove the darkness from the hair – this process is never temporary.

The lighteners are oxidising agents, usually hydrogen peroxide mixed with a setting lotion; these will gradually lighten the hair over a period of two to three days. On very dark hair the result would be an unsightly orange. If used regularly this will cause a regrowth.

Highlift tints
These are formulated to achieve a maximum lightening and tonal effect without bleaching. Best results are achieved on base shade above 6.

Mixing ratio is usually 1:2 using 40 vol/12% hydrogen peroxide.

Emulsion bleach
Emulsion bleaches are made up of three separate parts:
- an oil or gel bleach (ammonium hydroxide solution)
- hydrogen peroxide (normally 20 vol (6%) or 30 vol (9%))
- **boosters** or activators (sachets of powder).

Boosters are sometimes added to bleach products or lighteners to increase the amount of available oxygen, which increases the efficiency of the bleach or lightening product.

Always check the manufacturer's instructions for the recommended strength of peroxide and the number of boosters or activators to use.

Make sure you mix up in the correct order. The peroxide and boosters are generally mixed first and then the oil or gel bleach is added so that it does not become lumpy.

Emulsion bleaches are particularly good for whole-head and regrowth bleaches as the consistency is easy to apply.

TO DO

Look at the emulsion bleach left in the bowl after it has been used and see how much it has expanded due to the release of oxygen.

REMEMBER

If either the emulsion or powder bleach is coloured blue then it is difficult to see the correct degree of lightness. This is because the silver/blue colour neutralises the yellow/ orange colour of the bleached hair. You might therefore take the bleach off too soon, leaving the client with yellow (rather than light blonde) hair.
Always wash off the blue bleach with dampened cotton wool and check the colour by holding it over another piece of white cotton wool.

Powder bleach

Powder bleaches are made up of two parts:
- bleach powder (ammonium carbonate)
- hydrogen peroxide (normally 20 vol (6%) or 30 vol (9%)).

Powder bleaches have to be mixed to a smooth paste, but check the manufacturer's instructions as the amount of peroxide will vary if you are using liquid, as opposed to cream, peroxide.

Powder bleaches are also strong bleaches and are generally used for highlights and fashion effects. However, they do have a tendency to dry out and become powdery if excessive heat is applied.

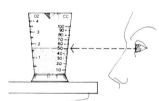

Measuring bleach

Always measure, check and mix bleach products carefully, checking the manufacturer's instructions. If you use peroxide that is too strong or mixtures of bleach that are too thick, you could burn the client's scalp and give an uneven colour to the hair. Peroxide that is too weak and bleach mixtures that are too thin can run into the client's eyes, skin and clothes, and will not lighten the hair enough.

The chemistry of bleaching

All bleaches are alkaline and contain ammonia (you can smell this quite strongly when mixing bleaches).

The alkali in bleaches has two actions:
- it swells the hair and opens up the cuticle scales so that the bleach can enter the cortex and lighten the colour pigments
- it mixes with the hydrogen peroxide (releasing the acid stabiliser in the peroxide) and releases the oxygen, which will bleach out the colour.

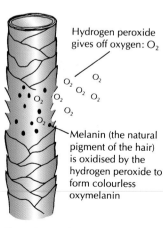

Hydrogen peroxide gives off oxygen: O_2

Melanin (the natural pigment of the hair) is oxidised by the hydrogen peroxide to form colourless oxymelanin

Changing melanin to oxymelanin

Nascent oxygen is newly formed oxygen. Unlike atmospheric oxygen, this has a powerful lightening effect on hair colour.

coloured pigment + nascent oxygen = oxy-pigment
(in the hair) (from hydrogen peroxide) (colourless)

This mixture works on the melanin and pheomelanin, resulting in oxidised pigment, which is colourless; this results in permanently lighter-coloured hair.
Hair when bleached will always lighten in this order:

black
dark brown
medium red brown
light warm brown
light golden brown
medium golden blonde
light blonde
very light blonde
white (disintegration).

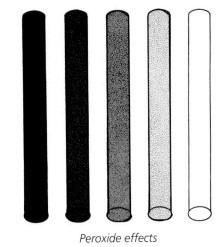

Peroxide effects

Hair must *never* be allowed to lighten beyond a very light blonde colour or it will disintegrate completely.

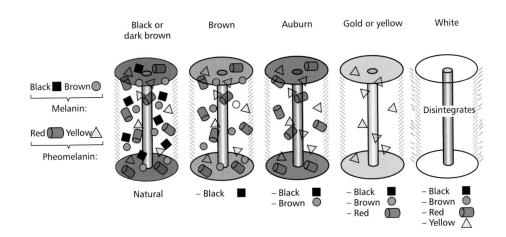

Bleaching out colour pigments

The swimming pool and ball and bleaching out colour pigment analogy

Removing colour pigments from hair is rather like trying to remove lots of balls from a swimming pool. Imagine that you are throwing in:

- six large black beach balls (black melanin pigments)
- 12 brown footballs (brown melanin pigments)
- five buckets of red tennis balls (red pheomelanin pigments)
- 10 buckets of yellow marbles (yellow pheomelanin pigments).

The large black balls in the pool would be easy to remove. The brown balls would take a little longer but would still be easy to pick up. This is similar to the black and brown melanin pigments lifting easily out of the hair. However, the red balls would take longer to retrieve – in the same way, when the hair turns red and orange during bleaching it takes a longer time to lift out. Lastly, lots and lots of small yellow balls would take a considerable time to pull out of the swimming pool. This is the same as the yellow pheomelanin pigment, which is the most difficult and slowest pigment to be removed from the hair.

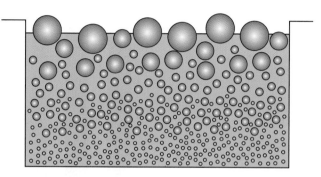

Swimming pool ball analogy

Bleaching removes melanin and pheomelanin in the following order.

PIGMENT COLOUR	BASE SHADE	DEPTH NUMBER
Black/brown	Black	1
	Very dark brown	2
	Dark brown	3
	Brown	4
Red/orange	Light brown	5
	Dark blonde	6
	Blonde	7
Orange/yellow	Blonde	7
	Light blonde	8
	Very light blonde	9
Yellow	Very light blonde	9
	Lightest blonde	10

TO DO

● *Take two test cuttings of naturally dark coloured hair. Bleach one of them with a little emulsion bleach, the other with a little powder bleach and 30 vol (9%) hydrogen peroxide, in a bowl.*

● *Watch the development very carefully, wiping the bleach off every 10 minutes to see all the warm orange and yellow colours produced before the hair becomes blonde.*

Application methods

Hair may be lightened with highlift tint (mixed with special developers), emulsion bleach or powder bleach, depending on the client's natural base shade and the degree of lift required. Generally, dark hair will need the stronger bleach products to lift. If in any doubt, take a test cutting.

Because of the danger of scalp burns it is advisable to use a maximum of 30 vol/9% 'on the scalp' (40 vol/12% is a recommended maximum for 'off the scalp').

The bleach must be applied evenly and with speed and accuracy to achieve an even lightening result.

Whole-head application

Both whole-head and regrowth bleaches are usually applied to hair sectioned into four as shown in the diagram.

Bleach is usually applied to the nape or crown area first where the hair is more resistant. Always apply bleach to a whole head of virgin hair in this order:
1 mid-lengths
2 ends of the hair
3 roots of the hair.

This is because the client's body heat (from the scalp) will make the bleach take more quickly near the scalp.

Never skimp with the amount of bleach. Take very small sections and always check the application thoroughly. The smallest area left uncovered will show up disastrously.

Regrowth application

When applying bleach to regrowth, you must always be thorough and never overlap on to the previously bleached hair, as hair breakage could occur.

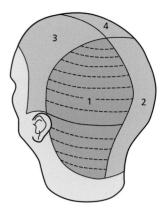
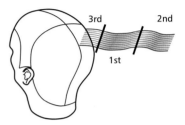

The four hair divisions

Whole-head application

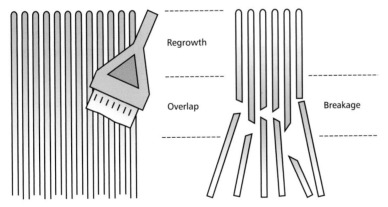
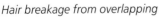

Hair breakage from overlapping

Checking the application

You can never be too careful when applying bleach. Always check the application from the opposite direction to the one in which you applied it.

If you have missed any areas, apply bleach to them immediately or dark patches will be seen. Pay special attention to the hairline and the thickest part of the hair (i.e. behind the ears).

Highlighting

This is a fashionable form of hair colouring. The hair is coloured to lighter shades. It involves separating strands of hair using a cap, plastic strips, foil or a spatula, and highlighting. Various shades can be used at one time on the various strands.

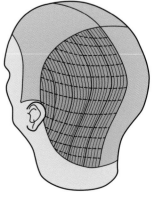

Cross-checking the application

Highlights also have the advantage that none of the product touches the scalp, which is useful for clients with sensitive scalps.

The cap method

Always brush the hair thoroughly in the direction of the style before putting on the cap. This will ensure that the highlights show in the correct areas of hair. Sometimes it is painful for the client when the highlight cap is put on, as it must be fixed securely and as close to the scalp as possible. A little talcum powder sprinkled inside the cap will make it easier to pull on.

Pull strands of hair through the cap using a highlight hook. Start pulling the strands through from the edges of the cap first to check the required thickness. This way, if the strands are too thick, they can easily be pulled back under the cap again with the highlight hook.

This is then combed to prevent the hair looping and to achieve full hair-length coverage.

Then mix the colouring product and apply to the strands using a brush. The hair is left to develop as per manufacturers' instructions. The cap may be covered to prevent the colouring product from drying out.

The advantage of this method is that it is very quick and easy, and it is ideally suited for short hair.

Woven highlights

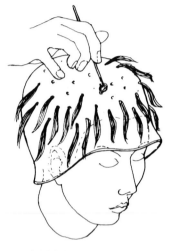

Cap highlights

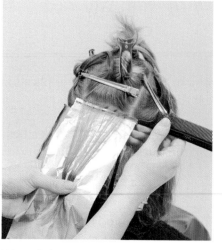

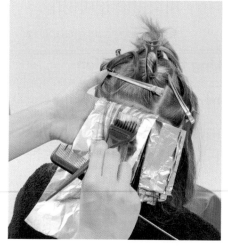

Preparing foil highlights　　　　*Weave hair*　　　　　　　*Apply product*

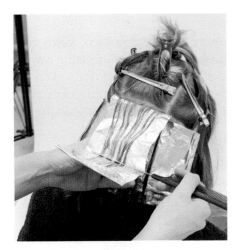

Fold foil lengthways

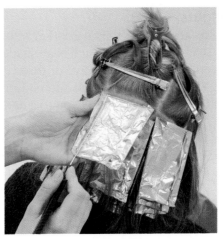

Complete parcel

These are used to separate and retain heat in the hair during processing.

Woven highlights are done with either foil or 'Easi-Meche' strips. Preparing woven highlights is a highly skilled technique.

Prepare the hair by sectioning in the 'nine-section' method (described in Chapter 9), so that you can work methodically, step by step.

Take sub-sections of hair of a similar size to those used for perming, and weave out the hair from the top of the section close to the scalp with a pin-tail comb. Place the woven strands on to the correct length of foil or Easi-Meche; apply bleach.

The foil or strip is then folded over the hair to form a packet and the root end should be surrounded closely to prevent unwanted leakage of the colouring product. Care must be taken not to overload the packet either with too much hair, as it could restrict the colouring effect, or too much colour, as seepage could occur.

Always start from the nape and work upwards.

When weaving out the strands of hair, always check that the strand directly below is woven, or the client will end up with stripes. As this is a lengthy process, some of the highlights may have developed to the required degree of lightness before completion, so check the development continually. If some highlights are ready, then stop the development on those strands only with cotton wool and warm water. To prevent this, use a lower-volume peroxide when you start mixing and a higher-volume peroxide towards the end of the technique; this will help all the highlights process at an even rate.

You might have to re-mix some fresh bleach if it takes you a long time (over 45 minutes) to complete the head, as the bleach mixture loses its strength after a time.

The advantages of woven highlights are that they are more comfortable for the client, you can see exactly where the highlights are being placed, you can mix tint and bleach highlights, and the product can be applied closer to the root area than with the cap method.

TO DO

Practise woven highlights on models who can spare the time, using thick conditioning cream instead of bleach.

REMEMBER

Always check that the length of foil is cut long enough for the length of hair.

Lowlights

Lowlights are colours that are darker or have more tone (e.g. golden, warm, red or silver) than the client's natural base shade. These are applied in the same way as cap or woven highlights. Often two or three colours are used together for woven highlights to give many varied and natural effects. For instance, gold, copper and light red colours woven alternately on to a dark blonde base can look particularly good.

Clients who have a lot of white hair around the front hairline may prefer a colour that matches their base shade woven into the white hair. This will blend the colour in and regrowth won't be so obvious when the hair grows out.

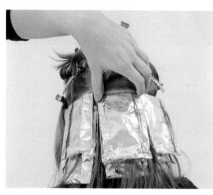
Bleach highlights with foil

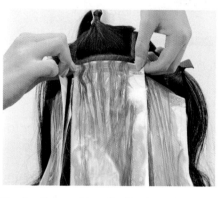
Tint lowlights with self-adhesive strips

Checking and timing the bleach

Apart from checking that you have not missed any areas of hair with the bleach, always make sure that no bleach has spilt on to the client's skin. If it has, remove it immediately with a dampened piece of cotton wool.

Time the bleach according to the manufacturer's instructions, but remember to test at frequent intervals because all bleaches have a variable development time, unlike tints, which have a set development time.

Testing

To test whether the bleach is ready, wipe the product from the hair with damp cotton wool and water. Then lay the strand over another piece of dry cotton wool so that you can see the true colour.

Hairdressers often do an elasticity test (sometimes called a tensile strength test) at this stage, using their fingers to test the amount of elasticity in the hair.

Removing the bleach

Whole-head or regrowth bleach

Remove the bleach product by rinsing thoroughly until the water runs clear. Use a lower water temperature than usual because the client's scalp will be sensitive, but ask the client if the temperature is comfortable.

Then gently shampoo the hair. If a bleach toner is to be used then do not use a conditioner, otherwise use an acid anti-oxy conditioner to return the hair to its natural acid state and close the cuticle scales.

REMEMBER

A warm salon will make the bleach take quicker. A cold salon will slow down the bleaching process.

Use any waiting time to clear up and write up your record card.

REMEMBER

Always check with your supervisor that you have chosen the proper correction to match the fault beforehand.

FAULT	CAUSES	CORRECTION
Hair damage/breakage	Applying bleach (overlapping) on to previously bleached hair	Recondition the hair and apply restructurants
	Incorrect proportions of mixture or too many boosters/activators used	
	Too high a concentration of hydrogen peroxide used	
	Over-developing the bleach, leaving it on too long (often due to not taking a strand test)	
	Processing with too much heat	
Skin/scalp damage	Not using barrier cream around the hairline	If just a little sore, then apply a soothing moisturising cream
	Use of too strong a bleach	If very inflamed, seek medical attention
	Over-developing the bleach: leaving it on too long	
	Cuts and abrasions on the scalp before bleaching	
Hair not light enough (i.e. too yellow)	Client's base colour too dark for the strength of bleach mixture used	Test hair elasticity and porosity; if satisfactory then re-bleach
	Bleach mixture too weak: peroxide strength too low	Apply a silver, ash or matt toner (for yellow, orange or red hair tones)
	Insufficient development time: bleach not left on long enough	Test hair for elasticity and porosity; if satisfactory then apply a silver, ash or matt toner (for yellow, orange or red hair tones)
Hair over-lightened	Use of too strong a bleach mixture	Recondition the hair, apply restructurants
	Over-developing the bleach: leaving it on too long	Re-colour under supervision
Uneven colour result	Uneven application	Spot bleach darker areas and re-bleach if under-processed
	Overlapping	
	No allowance made for body heat on a whole-head application	
	Bleach mixed badly, lumps left in the mixture	
	Sections too large	
	Application too slow	
	Seepage of product out of foils/meche	

Woven highlights

Carefully remove the tin foil or meche from the hair, then proceed as for a whole-head or regrowth bleach (above).

Cap highlights

Rinse the bleach from the highlights then use either a little shampoo or conditioner. Gently ease off the cap then proceed as for a whole-head or regrowth bleach (above). Finally, in all cases, complete the record card.

TEST YOUR KNOWLEDGE

1 What is the difference between highlights and lowlights?

2 List all of the tools and equipment available for highlighting or lowlighting hair and state how they are used.

3 What effect does a warm salon have on the bleaching process?

4 How does the client's body heat affect bleach development, and why is it important to keep checking on a bleach application?

5 Name two effects that hydrogen peroxide would have on hair if it were used by itself.

6 What is always released from hydrogen peroxide when it is mixed with bleaching products?

7 Which part of the hair is affected by bleach mixtures?

8 Why are bleaches always alkaline?

9 List the causes and corrections of the following problems:

  ● hair damage/breakage

  ● skin/scalp damage

  ● hair not light enough

  ● hair over-lightened

  ● uneven colour result.

10 What are your responsibilities to your client under the COSHH Act?

11 Why should you check with your supervisor if you are unsure about how to correct any mistakes?

Colour reducers

Colour reducers or colour strippers are used to remove permanent tints from the hair instead of using bleach.

They may be mixed with either water or peroxide, according to the desired result. Always check the manufacturer's instructions for mixing, application method and development time as these vary from one manufacturer to another.

The reducers work by breaking down the large dye molecules (which form tint colours permanently inside the cortex) into small dye molecules. These are then washed out of the hair after development time. This effectively reverses the dye process.

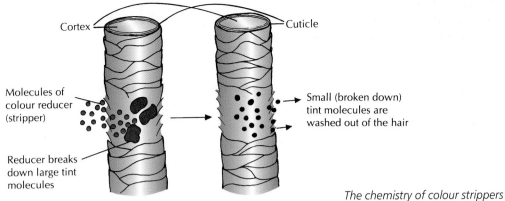

Cortex

Cuticle

Molecules of colour reducer (stripper)

Reducer breaks down large tint molecules

Small (broken down) tint molecules are washed out of the hair

The chemistry of colour strippers

Colour does not always strip easily out of the hair and often leaves the hair an uneven colour. A second application of colour stripper is often necessary to achieve an even colour, and a tint should always be applied afterwards to improve the final result.

Darkening bleached/lightened hair

Pre-pigmentation or colour filling is a technique used to compensate for the loss of yellow, orange and red pigments from bleached or lightened porous hair.

If this is not done when returning bleached or lightened hair to the client's natural base colour the result will be green or ashen.

There are several techniques to choose from.

- Use a semi-permanent yellow, orange or red colour first. Shampoo the hair, towel dry it, apply the semi-permanent colour, develop it, then blot off any excess with cotton wool. Apply one shade lighter than the required base colour tint mixed with peroxide directly over the top of the semi-permanent colour. Develop as normal.

- Use a permanent yellow, orange or red tone first. Do not use any peroxide. Apply it to dry hair, then blot off any excess with cotton wool. Apply one shade lighter than the required base colour tint mixed with peroxide directly over the top. Develop as normal.

- Use a permanent tint and peroxide, one shade lighter than the required base colour with a strong yellow, orange or red tone. Develop as normal.

Pre-pigmentation chart

ICC COLOUR DEPTHS		BLEACHED COLOUR TONES	PRE-PIGMENTATION COLOUR TONES NEEDED
10	Lightest blonde	Very pale yellow	
9	Very light blonde	Pale yellow	Yellow (golden)
8	Light blonde	Yellow	Yellow (golden)
7	Blonde	Orange-yellow	$\frac{3}{4}$ yellow (pale golden), $\frac{1}{4}$ orange (copper)
6	Dark blonde	Orange	$\frac{1}{2}$ yellow (golden), $\frac{1}{2}$ orange (copper)
5	Light brown	Reddish orange	Orange (copper)
4	Brown	Reddish brown	Red
3	Dark brown	Brown	Red
2	Very dark brown	Dark brown	Red
1	Black	Black	Red

TO DO

Check your salon's time allocations for the application of:
- *temporary colours*
- *semi-permanent colours*
- *quasi-permanent colours*
- *permanent colours – regrowth and full head*
- *lightening products/bleaches – regrowth and full head*
- *cap highlights*
- *foil highlights.*

Safety points to remember when colouring or bleaching

- Always read, check and follow the manufacturer's instructions. Measure all colouring products accurately.
- Make sure you have completed any necessary tests, such as porosity tests, elasticity tests, incompatibility tests, skin tests or test cuttings, before you start.
- Always agree the final colour with your client before starting.
- Gown up thoroughly so that no colour or bleach can stain the client's clothes.
- Apply barrier cream carefully to the client's hairline (but not their hair) before tinting or bleaching.
- Wear protective gloves when applying all bleaches and colourants.
- If you spill any products, clean up immediately.
- Complete and file record cards immediately after use.

TO DO

Re-read the section in Chapter 3 on the disposal of waste materials.

TEST YOUR KNOWLEDGE

1 State how the client's natural hair colour, depth and tone will affect the permanent colour result.
2 List the forms of tint available from various manufacturers.
3 Describe the effects of using different volumes of hydrogen peroxide for mixing with para tints.
4 What effect does a cold salon have on the tinting process?
5 How does body heat affect the application of a whole-head tint?
6 When would hydrogen peroxide be used by itself during tinting?
7 Which part of the hair is affected by para tints?
8 How do para tints work chemically on the hair?
9 How long should a permanent tint or a lightening product last on the hair?
10 Describe the effect of applying para tint to unevenly porous, highly sensitised hair (include any necessary precautions).
11 List the causes and corrections of the following problems:
   - colour too light
   - colour too dark
   - insufficient coverage
   - patchy, uneven results
   - skin staining.
12 What are your responsibilities to your client under the COSHH Act?
13 Why should you check with your supervisor if you are unsure about how to correct any mistakes?
14 How and why should waste be disposed of correctly?

Glossary

Accelerator: electrical equipment used to speed up a chemical process, uses infrared or radiated heat.

Acid: chemical with a pH of below 7.0, containing hydrogen ions.

Acid conditioner: acidic-based conditioner that helps restore the hair's pH balance.

Activator: substance that promotes activity.

Aescalup scissors: bulk-removing scissors. Also known as *thinning scissors*.

AIDS: acquired immune deficiency syndrome – a viral disease that attacks the immune system.

Air flow: stream of air from a hand-held hairdryer.

Alkaline: chemical with a pH of above 7.0, containing hydroxide ions.

Allergy: unpleasant reaction to a substance or chemical.

Alopecia: scientific name for baldness.

Alpha keratin: unstretched keratin hair shape.

Amino acid: small molecule that makes up the structure of keratin (hair).

Ammonium carbonate: active ingredient in bleaches, allowing for the quick release of oxygen.

Ammonium hydroxide: an alkaline chemical used in bleaching and perms.

Ammonium thioglycollate: active ingredient in 'cold wave' perms and the 'no lye' chemical product used in hair relaxing.

Anagen: active hair growing stage.

Analysis: examination of the clients' hair before carrying out any service.

Anti-clockwise curl: direction of pin curl. Also known as counter-clockwise curl.

Anti-oxidant conditioner: an acid based conditioner used to stop oxidation after a chemical process.

Antiseptic: a product that stops the growth of bacteria.

Arrector pili muscle: hair muscle connected to the hair and follicle.

Asymmetrical: unbalanced finish of a hairstyle.

Azo dyes: chemical used in temporary hair colours.

Back-brushing: brushing hair from ends to roots to add lift, volume and support to the hair.

Back-combing: combing hair from ends to roots to add lift, volume and support to the hair.

Backwash: washing basin where the client has to sit in a reclined position with the neck resting in the basin's recess.

Bacteria: rod-shaped or round micro-organisms.

Balance: a finished style with even proportions.

Baldness: hair condition that causes a lack of hair on the head.

Barber's itch: sycosis barbae – infectious skin disease affecting the beard area.

Barrel curl: a wide, stand-up curl with an open centre.

Barrelspring curl: curl formed in the shape of a barrel spring.

Barrier cream: thick waterproof cream that protects the skin from harsh chemicals.

Base shade: the natural colour of the hair.

Beta keratin: stretched keratin hair shape.

Bleach: a substance used to lighten hair colour.

Blonde: light-coloured brown or yellow hair.

Blood capillaries: tiny blood vessels that supply nutrients and oxygen to the hair.

Blow drying: styling and drying the hair using a hand dryer and a brush.

Blow waving: a technique that produces waves in the hair using a hand-held dryer and a comb or brush.

Blunt cut: club cut.

Booster: persulphate chemical that releases extra oxygen, used in bleaching.

Braid: plaited hair.

Brightening shampoo: a shampoo with mild lightening properties.

Buckled ends: fishhooks.

Cape: a covering for the client to protect their clothes.

Catagen: the second stage where hair slows down/stops growing.

Caucasian hair: European hair, usually straight or wavy.

Chipping-in: texturised hair-cutting technique.

Client: a customer of the salon.

Clientele: a group of customers of the salon.

Clippers: electrical or mechanical hair-cutting tool that club cuts the hair.

Clockspring curl: curl formed in the shape of a clockspring, with no centre.

Clockwise curl: a curl with its stem movements in the same direction as a moving clock.

Club cut: to cut hair that produces level ends.

Coarse hair: thick hair.

Cohesive set: technique of styling the hair by wetting, moulding and drying the hair.

Colour reducer/stripper: colour stripper, product that removes synthetic hair colour.

Colour shampoo: temporary colour, consists of a shampoo with colour added.

Colour star/circle: position of primary colours that are mixed together to make secondary colours, and are also opposite to each other.

Comb: tool with teeth used to style and dress hair.

Compound colours: combination of vegetable and mineral colours.

Conditioner: a product that corrects and improves the hair quality.

Contagious: infection caused by direct contact.

Contraindication: something that stops a service being performed.

Cool tones: blue, violet, green.

Cortex: central layer of hair, made from a collection of fibres, main structure of the hair.

Cowlick: strong hair growth pattern, on the front hairline.

Crest: the ridge or raised part of a wave.

Crimping: a method of adding fine wavy texture to hair.

Croquinole: method of winding hair from ends to roots.

Cross-linkages: chains that bond amino acids in the hair fibres.

Crown: upper area of the head.

Curl: rounded hair section.

Curler: roller or rod used to curl hair.

Curly hair: natural hair that has a lot of curl movement.

Cuticle: top or outer layer of the hair, made up of scales that look like fish scales or tiles on a roof.

Cutting angle: angle at which the hair is held and cut across the hair.

Cysteine: an amino acid with one sulphur atom made from a changed cystine molecule.

Cystine: an amino acid with a disulphide bond that is contained in hair.

Damaged hair: brittle, dry, split, non-elastic, porous hair.

Dandruff: pityriasis capitis – a scalp condition caused by the over-production of skin scales.

Delivery note: information written on paper that details what has been delivered by the supplier.

Demarcation: the line between the chemically processed hair and the regrowth.

Dense hair: thick or abundant hair.

Depilatory: an alkaline substance with a high pH value that is capable of dissolving hair.

Depth: the lightness or darkness of hair colour.

Dermal papilla: the group of cells at the base of the follicle that are the basis of hair growth.

Dermatitis: non-infectious skin condition caused by the skin's reaction to chemicals.

Dermis: known as the true skin, found under the epidermis.

Detergent: surface-active substance that cleans.

Development time: processing time.

Dilute: to thin down with a liquid.

Dirt: something that has germs.

Disease: illness of the mind or body.

Disentangle: to remove tangles and small knots.

Disinfectant: a substance capable of killing germs.

Disulphide bonds: two sulphur atoms in the hair that make very strong, non-water breakable cross-linkages.

Dressing: method of combing or brushing hair into a style.

Dry hair: hair that is not coated by sebum, making it feel rough, brittle and without shine.

Dryer attachment: a nozzle, diffuser or comb that fits on to a hand-held dryer and directs heated air flow.

Eccrine gland: sweat gland.

Eczema: non-infectious skin inflammation.

Effleurage: stroking hand massage movement, used to apply products.

Elasticity: the hair's ability to stretch and return to its original length.

Emulsify: to mix oil with water. Adding of water to a tint and massaging to loosen the tint from the hair and skin.

End paper: thin tissue used to prevent fishhooks while winding.

Epidermis: top surface of the skin.

European hair: Caucasian hair.

Face shape: the inside shape of the face.

Fading: short, graduated hair-cutting technique used in African Caribbean barbering.

Fashion colour: a well-liked colour that is in demand.

Feathering: to taper the hair ends using scissors.

Fine hair: thin hair with a small diameter.

Finger wave: moulded hair shapes formed into waves with the fingers and a comb.

Fishhook: distorted hair with bent backward hair ends caused by incorrect winding.

Foil: thin metallic sheet, used in hairdressing to wrap hair meshes.

Follicle: the 'pit' from which the hair grows.

Folliculitis: bacterial infection in the hair follicle.

Fragilitis crinium: split ends – hair is torn and brittle on the ends.

Frizz: hair with unwanted, very tight curls.

Fungi: plant organism.

Graduation: hair cut with shorter length at the nape, gradually lengthening towards the crown.

Grey hair: white hair reflecting coloured hair when mixed, giving the illusion of grey-coloured hair.

Guide line: first cut mesh of hair that is used as a guide for the rest of the haircut.

Hair: hardened strands of keratin that covers areas of the body.

Hair colour restorers: colours that contain metallic salts. Also known as *progressive dyes*.

Hair colouring: to add artificial colour to the hair.

Hair cut: hair shaping – a service that removes hair from the head.

Hair growth cycle: the three stages of hair growth: anagen, catagen and telogen.

Hairline: where the hair begins to grow on the edge of the scalp.

Hair papilla: base of the follicle where the hair grows.

Hairpins: fine pins use to secure curls and hair.

Hair relaxing: permanent process of straightening hair.

Hair shaft: hair that sticks out of the follicle.

Hairspray: finishing product used to hold a hairstyle in place.

Hairstyle: the finished look of the hair after dressing.

Hand-held dryer: a hairdryer held in the hand.

Head lice: parasite infestation, very contagious.

Head shape: the outer shape of the head.

Henna: Lawsone plant that is used in natural hair colouring.

High-frequency machine: equipment that uses electrical currents in its treatments.

Hollow-ground razor: a razor with concave shaped blade, e.g. German razor.

Honing: to edge set a razor blade using a hone or stone.

Hood dryer: a dryer the covers the head, used in wet setting.

Hot oil treatment: conditioning agent using warmed oil applied to the hair and scalp.

Humidity: the amount of moisture in the atmosphere.

Hydrogen peroxide: (H_2O_2) oxidising agent used in neutralisers and hair colouring.

Hydrophilic: water-loving part of a shampoo molecule.

Hydrophobic: water-hating or grease-loving part of a shampoo molecule.

Hygroscopic: hair's ability to absorb moisture from the atmosphere.

Impetigo: bacterial infection of the skin.

Incompatible: mixture of substances that create an unwanted reaction.

Incompatibility test: identifies any unwanted/incompatible chemicals on the hair.

Infection: obtaining a disease without direct contact.

Infestation: collection of parasites living on the body.

Inflammation: body irritation, usually seen as redness of the skin.

Irritant: a chemical/substance that causes the skin to itch or inflame.

Itch mite: sarcoptes scabiei – tiny parasites that cause scabies.

Keratin: hard sulphur containing chemical protein that hair is made from.

Lanolin: sheep sebum – used to moisturise the skin and hair.

Lanugo hair: soft, downy hair on an unborn child.

Lawsone: vegetable plant hair colouring, usually called henna.

Layering: haircut that reduces the lengths at different areas on the head.

Lightening: to lift or lighten hair colour.

Limescale: hard, crusty deposits caused by hard water, usually found on the inside of taps and showerheads.

Lowlights: darker-coloured streaks added to the hair.

Male pattern baldness: alopecia caused by a reaction to male hormones.

Marcel waving: waving hair using heated irons or tongs.

Massage: kneading, rubbing and stroking movements applied to the body to increase circulation.

Medulla: central part of the hair made of air spaces, not always present in the hair or along the length of the hair shaft.

Melanin: natural black/brown hair colour pigment molecules.

Mesh: small, manageable section of hair.

Micro-organism: a tiny living body.

Modern hair shaper: a razor with a safety guard and replaceable blades.

Molton Browners: long, flexible foam rollers used to curl the hair.

Monilethrix: condition that causes a beaded hair shaft.

Mongoloid hair: Asian hair – usually very straight.

Mousse: styling or colouring foam-producing product used in hairdressing services.

Nape: back of head joining the neck.

Natural movement: the natural way in which the hair lies.

Neck strip: a strip used around the neck to protect it; made of absorbent tissue.

Neutral: pH of 7.0, neither acid nor alkaline.

Neutralise: in perming: another name for fixing a curl in permanent waving; in colouring: to remove unwanted tones by applying the opposite colour.

Neutralising shampoo: specifically designed product to be used after the relaxing process to bring hair back to its natural pH scale.

Nit: egg of a pediculus capitis (head louse). Also known as *ova*.

Nitro dyes: chemicals used in semi-permanent hair colours.

Normalising: another name for neutralising.

Occipital bone: found at the back of the head above the nape line.

Open razor: a sharp blade with a handle, used to remove hair.

Overlap: incorrect application of chemical products being applied over previously chemical-treated hair, which can cause hair damage.

Over-process: to develop a chemical process for too long a time, causing hair damage.

Oxidiser/oxidant: product that releases oxygen.

Para dyes: chemicals used in permanent hair colours.

Parasite: a creature that lives off another living body.

Patch test: skin test.

Pathogenic bacteria: bacteria that cause disease.

Pediculosis capitis: invasion of the head by lice.

Penetrating conditioner: conditioner that is absorbed into the hair.

Permanent colour: hair colour that does not wash out and leaves a regrowth of natural colour as the hair grows.

Permanent wave: a curl made permanent by chemicals so it does not fall out.

Perming: method of curling/waving the hair permanently.

Petrissage: deep, circular hand massage movement, used to stimulate the scalp and relax the client.

pH scale: measurement of acid and alkaline substances.

Pheomelanin: natural red/yellow hair colour pigment molecules.

Pin curl: a curl secured with pins.

Plaiting: intertwining strands of hair.

Pleat: hairstyle that has a folded or rolled shape.

Pli: full French name *mise-en-pli*, meaning set hair.

Polypeptide chain: long chain molecules made from amino acids and cross-linked with disulphide bonds.

Porosity test: to test the hair's ability to absorb liquids, by checking cuticle damage.

Porous: hairs' ability to absorb moisture caused by opened cuticle scales.

Post-damp: where hair is wound before perm lotion is applied.

Postiche: wig or hairpiece made of hair.

Pre-damp: where perm lotion is applied during the winding process.

Pre-pigmentation: adding colours to the hair to replace lost pigments to enable another colour to develop.

Pre-soften: a process that lifts the cuticle scales for a chemical service by applying hydrogen peroxide.

Processing time: time given to develop colours and perms.

Professional: a learned person who acts with high standards.

Psoriasis: non-infectious skin disease.

Quasi-permanent: nearly, but not quite permanent hair colour. Also known as tone-on-tone, deposit-only, oxy-permanents.

Razor cutting: to remove hair using a razor.

Reception: place where clients are received.

Receptionist: trained person who deals with reception duties.

Record card: card containing information written about clients that details their services.

Reducing agent: product that enables the addition of hydrogen or the removal of oxygen.

Regrowth: new hair grown from the roots after a chemical process.

Relaxer: chemical product that removes curls or wave movement from the hair.

Request: a thing or service asked for.

Resistant hair: hair with tightly closed cuticle scales that resist chemical applications.

Retouch: to chemically process regrown hair only, either colour or perm.

Reverse graduation: hair cut with longer length at the nape, gradually shortening towards the crown.

Ringlet: a spiral curl that hangs downwards.

Ringworm: tinea capitis – infectious fungal skin disease.

Rod: tool used to curl hair in perming.

Rotary: quick, circular hand massage movement, used to cleanse.

Salt linkages: water-breakable bonds in the hair structure.

Scalp: skin and muscle that covers the top part of the head.

Scissors: a pair of edged blades with handles used to remove hair.

Scrunch dry: technique that dries the hair using the hands and a hand-held hair dryer.

Sebaceous gland: gland that produces sebum.

Sebum: natural oil made from the body, used to moisturise the skin and hair.

Sectioning: division of hair.

Set: to wind hair around rollers to create movement and volume.

Shampoo: a substance used to cleanse.

Skin test: to assess the skins' sensitivity to a tint.

Sodium bromate: oxidising agent used in neutralisers.

Sodium hydroxide: 'lye' chemical used in hair relaxing.

Solid razor: French razor, quieter to use than a hollow-ground razor.

Solvent: chemical substance that will dissolve another chemical.

Spiral curl: curls formed from winding roots to ends.

Split ends: fragilitis crinium – damaged, torn hair ends.

Stabiliser: acid-based chemical that helps hydrogen peroxide keep its strength.

Stand-up curl: curl stem sticking up from the head.

Static electricity: friction of combing or brushing causing 'flyaway' hair.

Steamer: electric hood equipment that produces moist heat.

Sterilise: to make free from germs.

Sterilising cabinet: a box that uses ultraviolet rays to sterilise tools.

Strand test: to assess the result or suitability of hair colouring.

Strop: a length of leather with a handle, used to smooth a razor's edge.

Substantive conditioner: conditioners that are able to enter the hair shaft easily.

Sulphur bonds: non-water breakable bonds that make up cross-linkages found in the polypeptide chains.

Surface conditioner: conditioner that coats the hair cuticle only.

Surface tension: thin, film-like layer on top of liquid surfaces.

Sweat gland: eccrine gland that produces sweat, the body's natural cooling agent.

Symmetrical: an evenly balanced hairstyle.

Synthetic: not natural, artificial, man-made.

Tail comb: comb with a long, thin handle used for lifting and sectioning hair.

Tease: to separate or lift small amounts of hair into place.

Telogen: hair growth in its resting stage.

Temporary colour: a surface colour that coats the cuticle scale; lasts until next shampoo.

Temporary curl: a curl that drops when it comes into contact with moisture.

Tensile strength: tension or pull put on hair to test its strength.

Tension: pulling pressure put on the hair, causing it to stretch.

Terminal hair: strong coloured coarse hairs found on scalp and on men's faces (beards).

Test curl: test to check the strength of a curl during permanent waving.

Test cutting: small cutting of hair with colour applied; used to check colour result and suitability before starting full colour service.

Texture: diameter of a hair shaft; it can be fine or coarse.

Thinning: to cut hair so the bulk of the hair is removed, and the length is retained.

Thinning scissors: a pair of scissors with one or both edge blades serrated.

Tinea capitis: ringworm on the scalp.

Tint gown: protective covering for the client.

Tinting: a service that applies colour, usually permanent, to the hair.

Tone: colour we actually see.

Towel dry: to remove excess water using a towel after washing hair .

Traction alopecia: hair loss caused by pulling hair out at its roots.

Translucent: see through; lets light pass through.

Trichology: study of the hair and scalp.

Trichohexis nodosa: swollen hair shaft caused by harsh physical and chemical damage.

Trim: haircut that removes very little length and retains the shape.

Ultraviolet rays: rays that can be used to sterilise tools. These rays are damaging to the eyes and skin.

Under-developed/processed: to develop a chemical process for too little time.

Uneven colour: hair colour that is patchy along the hair shaft.

Vellus hair: fine, downy hair found on the body and face; usually has no colour.

Ventilation: circulation of air.

Vibro massager: electrical massaging equipment.

Virgin hair: hair that has not been chemically processed.

Virus: smallest micro-organism that causes illness.

Volume: amount of hair on the head.

Warm tone: red and gold (yellow) and copper (orange).

Wave: loose curl or dressed shape.

Wet set: cohesive set.

Wetting agent: substance that lowers liquid surface tension allowing the liquid to cover more area.

Wig: false hair that covers the full head.

Winding: wrapping hair around a roller.

Zinc pyrithione: chemical contained in anti-dandruff shampoo.

Index

entries in **bold** also appear in the glossary pp. 263–8

barrier cream   5, 65, 93, 205, 212
base shade   232, 233, 234, 246, 254
basins   90
basing cream   213
beaded hair shaft (monilethrix)
   12, 13
beards   187, 195, 196
   cutting   195, 198, 199, 200
benefits, explaining   33, 34, 35,
   37, 80
beta keratin   118–19, 135, 136
bills, client   84
bleach   68, 71, 230, 260
   baths   244, 250
   blue   252
   boosters   251–2
   emulsion   251–2, 254
   toner   258
bleached hair, processing   202,
   261
bleaching   17, 236–8, 251–60, 262
   faults   259
   products   251
   safety points   262
bleeding   71, 110, 200
blood capillaries   8, 9, 105
blood pressure   111, 112
'blotting'   224
blow drying   117, 118–23, 126–9,
   130, 132
blow waving   128, 129
blue bleach   252
blunt (club, precision) cut   161,
   164, 168, 169, 185, 186
bobs   168, 169, 180
body build   19, 186
body language   36
bonds
   disulphide   7–8, 203, 213, 214,
      215, 224
   hydrogen   7, 118, 119, 132
   lanthionine   214
   temporary   118, 119, 135
bones of the head   107, 184
boosters, bleach   251–2

boosters, curl   212, 213
braids   149–50, 151, 153
'brassy' hair   240
breakage of hair   216, 221, 237, 259
brick winding   145, 209–10
brightening shampoo   244
brilliantines   131
brushes 120–1, 129, 137
   bristle (Denman)   121, 146, 187
   hot   124
   neck   188
   vent   120, 129, 146, 165, 187
brushing, bad   16
'bubbling'   126
buckled ends   154, 205, 221
build-up of products   98
burns   65, 71, 126
   pull   210–11, 221
   scalp and skin   206, 210, 255
butterfly clips   122, 165
buying signals   33

caffeine   109
calcium hydroxide (non-lye)   214,
   215, 217, 221
cancer   100
cap highlights   256, 260
cardiac arrest   69
careers   x, xi
catagen stage of growth   9
Caucasian hair   10, 157
caustic soda (lye)   214, 215, 217,
   221
checklists   28–9, 46
chemical bonds
   disulphide   7–8
   hydrogen   7, 118, 119, 132
chemical burns   65
chemical damage 16–17
chemicals
   in the eye   71
   hazardous   61–2, 63, 67, 68, 202
   relaxing   214–15, 217–18
   safety   67–8
   storing   67

friction massage 113, 194

frictions 131, 194

fringes 21, 161, 171, 176

frizz 16, 17, 130, 131, 148

fungus conditions 14, 54, 55, 112

gels 130, 136

gent's traditional cut 193

germicides 92

glossary 263–8

gloves, protective 206, 210

glyceryl monothioglycollate 204

'goose pimples' 8, 105

gowning up 5, 90, 155, 188, 197, 201

gowns 5, 56

graduated layer cut 166, 167, 173, 174–7, 179

greasy hair 13, 30, 95, 96, 102

Grecian 2000 23, 246

green hair 250, 261

grey hair 230–1, 242

groom 130

gross misconduct 74

growth of hair 9–10, 113, 181

  patterns 20–1, 118, 135, 148, 157, 184

    facial hair 196

hair mascara 241

hair nets 139

haircuts 181, 184

Hairdressing Manufacturers' and Wholesalers' Association (HMWA) 61, 62

hairdryers 114, 122–3, 132, 139, 207

hairgrips 139, 149

hairlines 164, 184, 185, 187, 188

hairpins 138

hairspray 119, 131, 136, 147, 241

hairstyles 17, 147, 169

Haringtons 169, 172, 173, 177

hazardous chemicals 61–2, 63, 67, 68, 202

hazards in the salon 65

head bones 107, 184

head lice (pediculosis capitis) 12, 14, 15, 54, 55, 112

head shape 17–18, 148, 184

Health and Safety at Work Act (HASAWA) 1974 61, 63, 68

Health and Safety Regulations 63

health matters

  back care 123, 129, 159

  exercise 59

  feet 58, 129

  lifting and carrying 41

  muscles 79, 109, 123, 159

  posture 57

  standing 1, 6, 90, 123

  wrist strain 58, 90, 159

heated rollers 144

height of client 19

henna (Lawsone) 246

hepatitis B 55, 71, 72, 180

high blood pressure (hypertension) 111, 112

highlift tints 230, 251, 254

highlights 230, 237, 251, 255–7, 258, 260

  foil 235, 256–7, 258

hood dryers 114, 139, 207

hormones 100, 102, 105, 185

hot brushes 124

hot oil treatment 102

humidity 68

hydrocortisone creams 109

hydrogen bonds 7, 118, 119, 132

hydrogen peroxide 24, 27, 65, 68, 223

  bleaching and colouring 236–8, 251

  dilutions and strengths 237, 238

  storage 237

hydrolysis 214

hygiene, personal 57

hygiene, salon 54, 55–6

hypersensitivity tests (skin tests) 27

hypertension (high blood pressure)   111, 112
hypochlorite   56
hypotension (low blood pressure)   111

immune system   106
impetigo (oozing pustules)   14, 15, 55
incompatibility test   23, 24
infectious conditions   12, 14–15, 54, 55, 112
infestations   14, 112
influenza (flu)   54
injury, personal   63
inside shapes   179
insulin   111
insurance   59
International Colour Chart System (ICC)   233, 234, 261
irritants   67, 68, 93

jewellery   57
job descriptions   47–8
job shadowing   51

keratin   7, 8, 9, 11, 13, 16, 99
   alpha and beta   118–19, 135, 136

lanolin   92
lanthionine bonds   214
lanugo hair   8
Lawsone   246
layered cuts   167, 170–7, 181, 183, 189, 190
legislation
   Acts   2, 42–4, 59–64, 68, 71, 77
   Regulations   59–60, 61, 62, 64
lemon juice   102
life cycle of hair   9–10
lifestyle of clients   3, 20
lifting   41
lighteners, temporary   251
limescale   91
lines of cut   178–9

lining out   164, 187, 188
liquid measures   238
long hair   104, 134, 143, 148–51, 175, 176
loss of hair   185
low blood pressure (hypotension)   111
lowlights   230, 234, 245, 258
lye (caustic soda)   214, 215, 217, 221
lymphatic system   106–7

male pattern baldness   13, 185
Management of Health and Safety at Work Regulations (MHSWR) 1999   63
Manual Handling Operations Regulations 1992   62
marcel waving irons   134
massage   106, 107, 112–13
   contraindications   110–12
   effleurage   97, 106, 112
   friction   113, 194
   head   97, 105
   machines for   113
   petrissage   112–13
   tapotement   113
   vibration   113
measuring liquids   238
medication   100, 109
medulla   6, 7, 8
melanin   6, 8, 10, 13, 231, 252–4
melanocytes   13
messages, telephone   82
metallic dyes   23, 24, 218, 246
micro-organisms   54
migraine   111
mirrors   139, 165
mites   14
moisturisers   131
moles   13
Molton Browners   138, 143
monilethrix (beaded hair shaft)   12, 13
Mongoloid (Asian) **hair**   10, 157